The 30-Minute
MIND Diet Cookbook

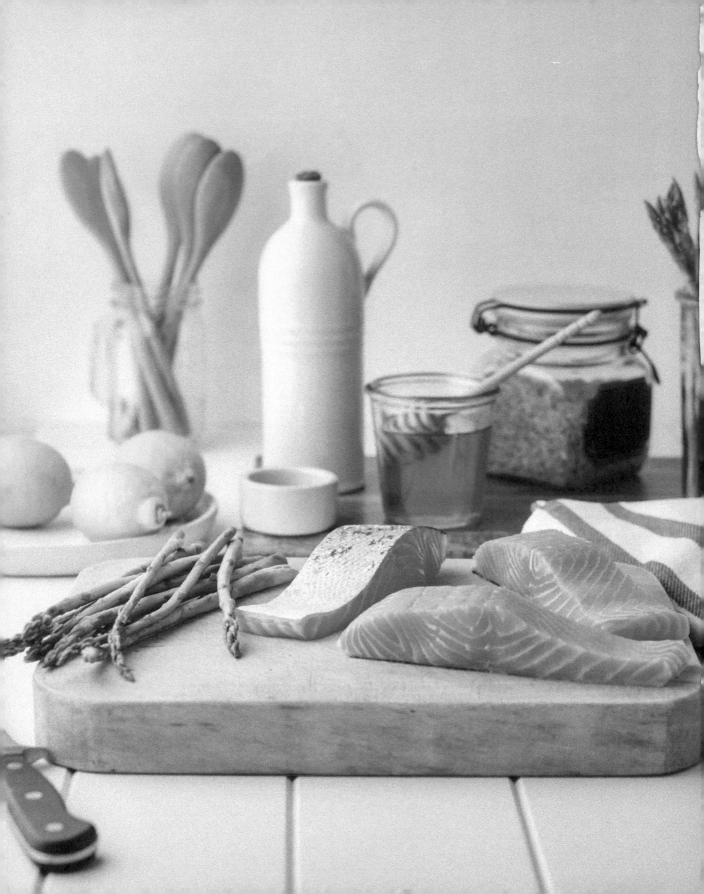

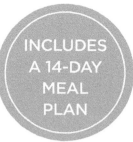

INCLUDES
A 14-DAY
MEAL
PLAN

the 30-minute
MIND*diet*
COOKBOOK

Recipes to Enhance
Brain Health and
Help Prevent Alzheimer's
and Dementia

Amanda Foote, RD

Photography by Darren Muir

**ROCKRIDGE
PRESS**

For general information on our other products and services or to obtain technical support, please contact our Customer Care Department within the United States at (866) 744-2665, or outside the United States at (510) 253-0500.

Rockridge Press publishes its books in a variety of electronic and print formats. Some content that appears in print may not be available in electronic books, and vice versa.

Interior and Cover Designer: Heather Krakora

Art Producer: Janice Ackerman
Associate Editor: Maxine Marshall
Production Editor: Mia Moran
Production Manager: Martin Worthington
Photography © 2021 Darren Muir. Food styling by Yolanda Muir
Author photo courtesy of Hardstep Design

ISBN: Print 978-1-64876-683-1 | eBook 978-1-64876-180-5

R0

For my Grandma, Jo

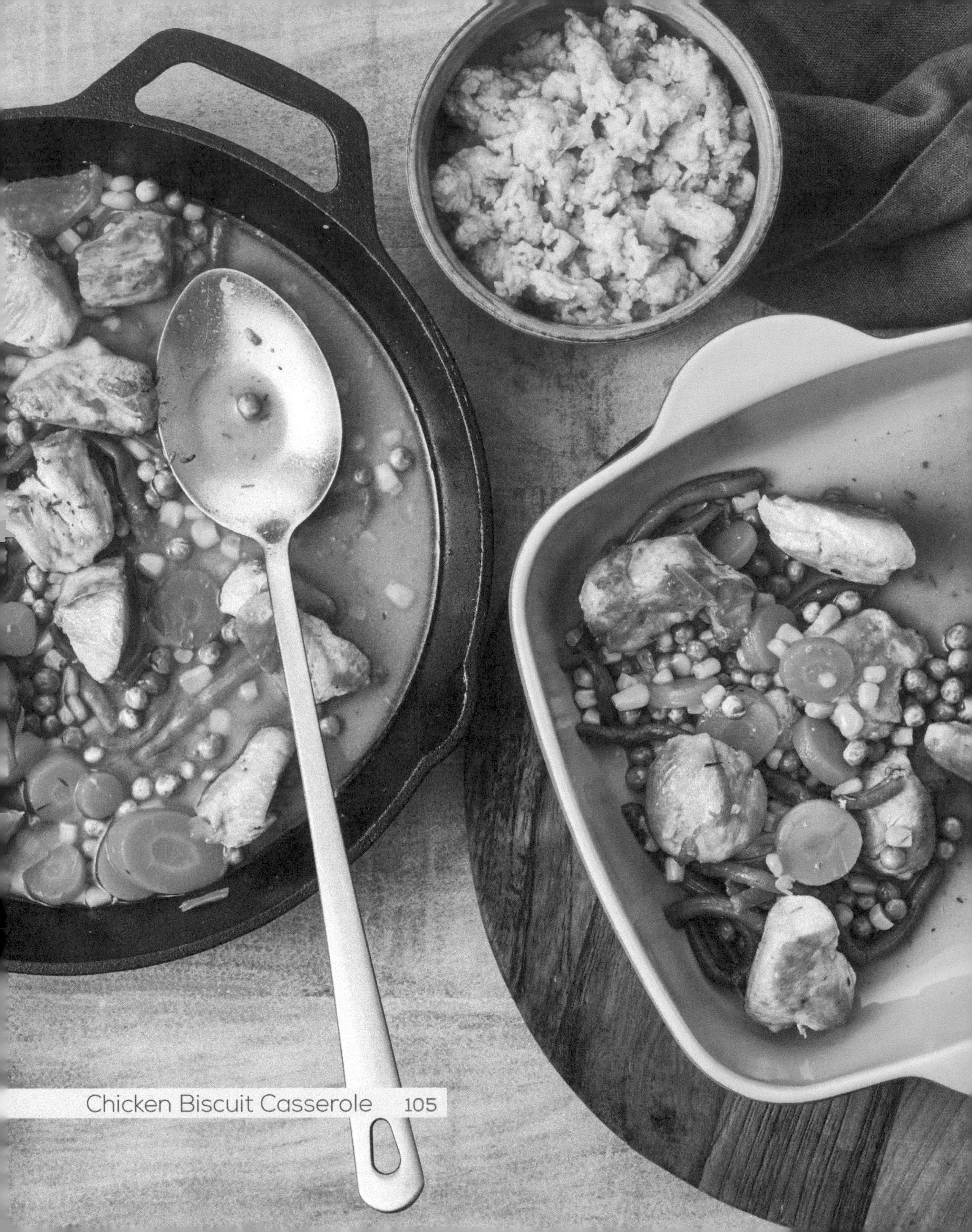

Chicken Biscuit Casserole

CONTENTS

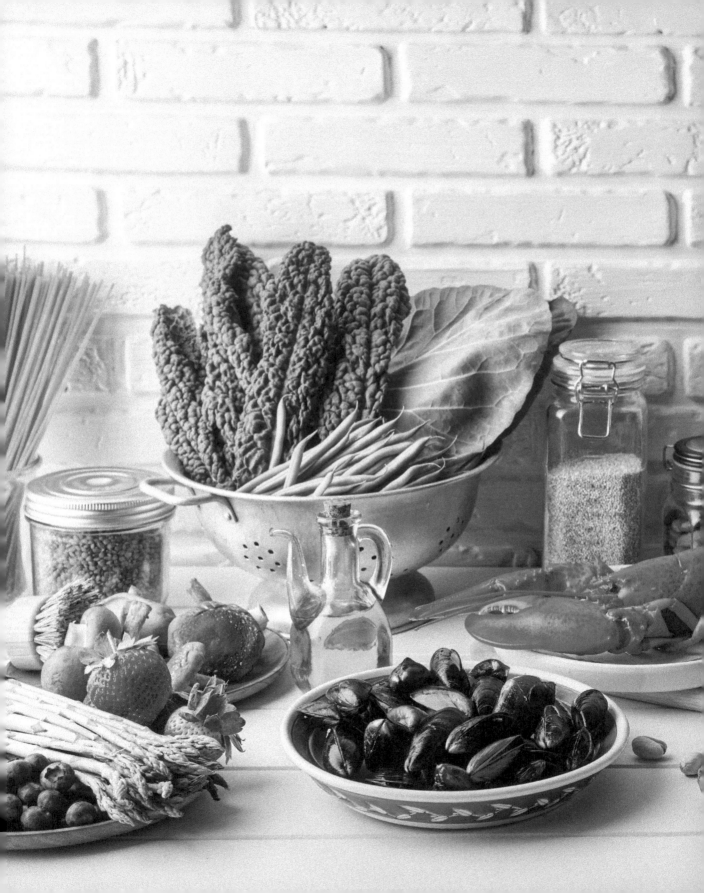

INTRODUCTION

Cognitive decline is a great concern as we grow older. Fortunately, our understanding of the causes of cognitive decline—and of preventive measures—has drastically changed in recent decades, offering an abundance of new hope. Nutrition has been proven to be an effective tool for disease prevention and management. Groundbreaking research by Harvard Medical School has proven that healthy lifestyle choices can prevent and treat cognitive decline. The MIND diet provides us a real opportunity to use food as medicine, and I am here to tell you that the "medicine" is going to be delicious. The recipes in this book include household favorites modified for brain health as well as new flavors for you to savor.

This journey is close to my heart. I am a registered dietitian with a passion for brain health. My dear grandmother lost her battle with dementia in 2019, so I deeply understand the importance of preventing and delaying the onset of Alzheimer's disease and dementia.

This book is for anyone, at any stage of life. Eating a brain-healthy diet can only benefit you, and it is never too early or late to start. You may be interested in the MIND diet because you have read about how important nutrition and lifestyle are for your future health. Or you may just be looking for simple, affordable, delicious meals that are ready in under 30 minutes, and the fact that they benefit brain health is an added bonus.

No matter who you are or where you are in life, I thank you for picking up a copy of my book, and I genuinely hope that you enjoy the recipes and that you live in good health. My wish is that you not only find a renewed joy for cooking and new recipes to add into your meal rotation but also discover just how easy, inexpensive, and tasty eating well for better brain health can be.

Welcome, and, please, let's dig in!

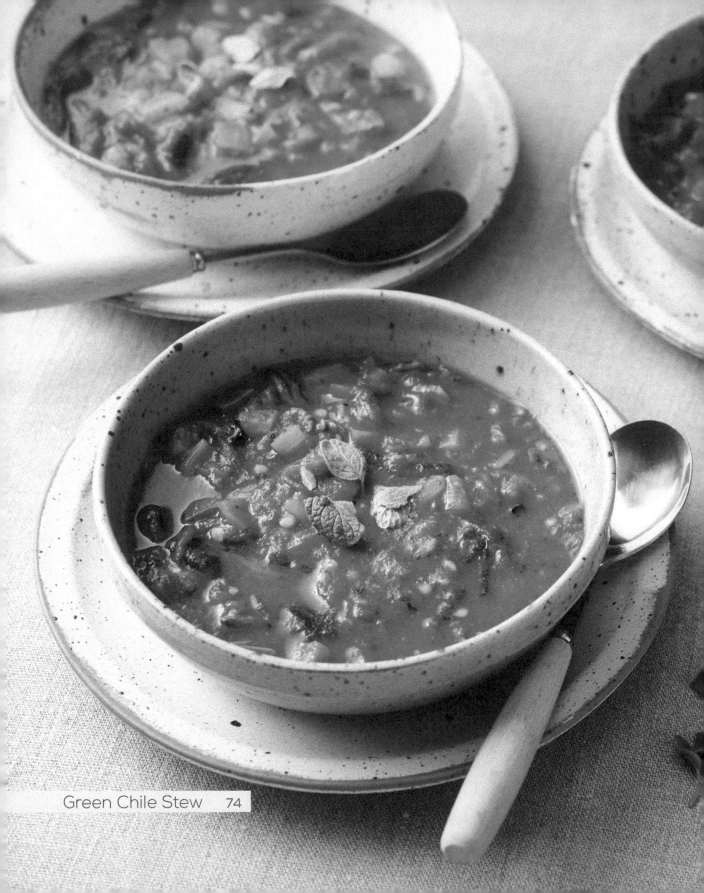

Green Chile Stew 74

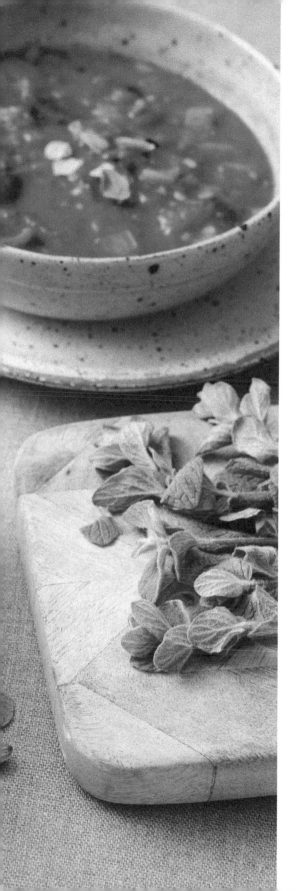

CHAPTER ONE

The MIND Diet Explained

Before we get into the delicious recipe goodness of this book, I'd like to first take a moment to talk about what the MIND diet is. With so many fad diets flying around, it is important for me to point out that the MIND diet is wholly based in science and is a dietary pattern, *not* a weight-loss "diet." We will dive into the science behind the MIND diet and the biology of Alzheimer's disease and dementia to discover how your food choices can positively benefit your brain.

What Is the MIND Diet?

The MIND diet was created by nutritional epidemiologist Dr. Martha Morris, combining the best elements of the Mediterranean diet and the Dietary Approaches to Stop Hypertension (DASH) diet. The MIND diet stands for:

Mediterranean-DASH
Intervention for
Neurodegenerative
Delay

The Mediterranean diet has been widely researched because people living in the Mediterranean region have comparatively low rates of cardiovascular disease–related death. The DASH diet was created by the National Institutes of Health to prevent high blood pressure. Both diets are rich in fruit, vegetables, whole grains, plant oils, lean poultry and fish, nuts, and seeds. Both diets limit red meat, which can be detrimental to cardiovascular health.

Putting all this amazing research into action, Dr. Morris found a balance between the two diets that can prevent or delay the onset of cognitive decline. At its core, the MIND diet promotes daily and weekly portions of vegetables, leafy greens, berries and other fruits, whole grains, nuts, olive oil, seafood, and red wine (if you choose and if your doctor approves your intake of alcohol). The MIND diet limits saturated and trans fats as well as added sugar.

While factors like genetics play a role in cognitive health, research on the MIND diet shows that it is never too early or late to benefit from a healthy diet to preserve your mind and overall health.

THE SCIENCE

Several studies have influenced the science around cognitive health, two of which are particularly monumental: the Chicago Health and Aging Project (CHAP) and the Memory and Aging Project (MAP).

CHAP evaluated over 10,000 seniors for three consecutive years to monitor their health, cognition, and lifestyle. The study found that diet has a significant impact on the incidence and development of Alzheimer's disease. It found that unsaturated fats, omega-3 fatty acids, and antioxidants lowered the risk of developing Alzheimer's disease.

MAP followed nearly 2,000 seniors with annual evaluations of cognition, diet, and other factors. The MAP participants all agreed to donate their brains for research after their deaths. Ongoing research on genetics and risk from environmental agents such as diet and lifestyle looks very promising. MAP is an active study, and we will continue to learn more about Alzheimer's disease and dementia from it.

These studies were fundamental in the creation of the MIND diet by Dr. Morris and Rush University Medical Center. Both studies identified diet as a central element that can cause or prevent Alzheimer's disease and dementia, with research finding that cognitive decline was reduced by the intake of antioxidants, B vitamins, flavonoids, carotenoids, polyphenols, omega-3 fatty acids, and unsaturated fats. And so, the MIND diet was born.

A subsequent 2015 study found that the MIND diet lowered the risk of Alzheimer's disease by up to 53 percent in participants who followed the diet strictly and by about 35 percent for those who followed it moderately well.

How Our Brains Can Change

Our brains change in several ways as we age. While some are a natural part of growing older, others can indicate more serious cognitive conditions.

NATURAL COGNITIVE AGING

According to the Alzheimer's Association, the older we get, the more difficulty we may have pulling up a memory, maintaining our train of thought, or even finding objects around the house. This is completely normal, and these occurrences usually do not significantly affect how people perform daily activities.

The next level of cognitive aging is known as mild cognitive impairment (MCI), which 15 to 20 percent of seniors experience after age 65. MCI affects memory and decision making. A person with MCI may have trouble remembering recent conversations or events or may experience difficulty in completing tasks. While MCI doesn't significantly interfere with the ability to perform daily activities, the difficulty is noticeable by friends and family. It does not always lead to a more serious cognitive condition, but a person with MCI is at higher risk for developing dementia or Alzheimer's disease.

DEMENTIA

Dementia is a condition that encompasses several more specific diseases, including Alzheimer's disease, Lewy body dementia, vascular dementia, frontotemporal dementia, Parkinson's disease, and Huntington's disease. Simply put, dementia involves abnormal brain changes that interfere with daily life. Symptoms can involve memory loss but also impair daily activities like eating, dressing, and bathing. A person with dementia may have difficulty with short-term memory, finding commonly used objects like keys, finding their way home, and managing finances. The Alzheimer's Association that estimates nearly 10 percent of people over the age of 60 have some form of dementia.

Although there is no known cure for dementia, medications and treatments can help improve quality of life by managing symptoms. Research is promising and has shown that diet and lifestyle changes can reduce the risk of developing dementia and can slow the onset.

ALZHEIMER'S DISEASE

Alzheimer's disease is a form of dementia that is most characterized by memory loss as well as an inability to learn new information and make sound decisions. As it becomes more severe, Alzheimer's disease may cause mood disturbances, behavior changes, paranoia, delusions, and physiological difficulties with speaking, moving, or even swallowing.

The Alzheimer's Association estimates that 10 percent of seniors over age 65 have some level of Alzheimer's disease. This is a normal pathology due to brain aging; over time, plaque accumulates around the neurons in the brain, causing a barrier to effective communication between the cells. Our neurons can also develop tangles, which further impairs the functioning of the cells. This information has come to us from groundbreaking research and technological advances in brain imaging. Doctors are now able to map the progression of Alzheimer's disease, thus revolutionizing how it is prevented and treated.

There is currently no cure for Alzheimer's disease, but there are treatments that may help improve the quality of life. What has become clearer in recent decades is that the MIND diet is an excellent tool for preventing Alzheimer's disease and slowing its progression in some cases. Nutrition is a proven way to improve brain health, keeping cells energized, flexible, and effective.

CONSIDERING THE RISK FACTORS

The biggest risk factors for cognitive decline include inflammation, oxidative stress, smoking, high blood pressure, diabetes, and high cholesterol. The best news is that you have the power to reduce your risk factors. If you'd like to explore more, Dr. Morris discusses these risk factors in depth in her body of research.

Inflammation is a broad term for when the body is trying to fight off illness, injury, or toxins. Inflammation is a positive protective bodily response, but when the source of the "danger" is constant, inflammation becomes chronic, and healthy tissues and systems are damaged. Poor diet, excess body fat, and smoking are all causes of inflammation.

Oxidative stress is caused by excess free radicals, which come from natural body processes as well as from diet and environmental pollutants. Free radicals are molecules the body produces when it breaks down food, pollutants, or tobacco smoke. Diets high in fatty animal products, added sugar, and highly processed foods are linked to oxidative stress.

Smoking increases the risk for all vascular diseases, including those of the brain, such as strokes and dementia. The toxins in tobacco alone cause both inflammation and oxidative stress.

High blood pressure can cause plaque accumulation in the brain, which narrows blood vessels. This narrowing is linked to the development of Alzheimer's disease. High blood pressure is often caused by diet and lifestyle choices, including consuming high-fat and salt-laden foods, not exercising sufficiently, and smoking.

Type 2 diabetes is highly correlated with Alzheimer's disease. A Mayo Clinic study found that 81 percent of patients with Alzheimer's disease had type 2 diabetes or impaired fasting glucose. Diabetes is not completely caused by lifestyle and diet, as there are biological and genetic predispositions. However, proper nutrition is an excellent tool for preventing and controlling diabetes, thereby preventing or delaying cognitive decline.

High LDL ("bad") cholesterol has been linked to early-onset Alzheimer's disease, as was demonstrated in a 2019 *JAMA Neurology* study. There are several genetic risk factors for high cholesterol, but it can also be caused by a high-fat diet.

How Diet Affects Your Brain

The amazing takeaway from all the research is that there is a link between what is on our plates and how our brains age. Let's unpack the main findings of MIND diet research regarding how diet and nutrients influence brain functioning. In the next chapter (see page 11), we'll look more closely at which foods to fill your plate with in order to reap the benefits of these nutrients.

FATS

Fat is an important energy source for the body, essential for cells to function. However, there are different kinds of fat and not all fat is created equal.

Saturated and trans fats are unhealthy fats that raise bad cholesterol and increase your risk of developing cardiovascular disease. The simplest way to identify unhealthy fats is that they are usually solid at room temperature. Some examples include bacon, butter, and lard.

Unsaturated fats decrease bad cholesterol and raise good cholesterol. Monounsaturated and polyunsaturated fats are found in plant oils, nuts, and avocados. Unlike saturated fats, unsaturated fats are primarily liquid at room temperature. Examples include olive oil, canola oil, and corn oil.

Omega-3 fatty acids, including alpha-linolenic acid (ALA) and docosahexaenoic acid (DHA), are specific polyunsaturated fats that are particularly effective at reducing your risk for cardiovascular disease and neurodegenerative disease. Omega-3 fatty acids are found in finfish, seafood, fish oil supplements, flaxseed oil, canola oil, nuts, and seeds.

VITAMIN E

Vitamin E is a crucial antioxidant that helps trap free radicals and thus prevent oxidative damage in the body. It also protects memory and brain function, helping reduce the risk of developing Alzheimer's disease. This is because vitamin E forms a layer around cells to protect them from oxidative stress. Studies have found that patients with Alzheimer's disease have lower levels of vitamin E in their bodies, which may have caused their neurons to experience damage from inflammation and oxidative stress. Vitamin E is found in nuts, seeds, and plant oils.

VITAMIN C

Vitamin C is another key nutrient because it helps vitamin E work even more effectively in the body. An antioxidant in its own right, vitamin C is a major player in countless biological functions that benefit overall brain health. Vitamin C is found in broccoli, Brussels sprouts, cantaloupes, citrus fruits, chiles, kale, parsley, strawberries, sweet peppers, and thyme.

B VITAMINS

B vitamins play a critical role in prevention of dementia and Alzheimer's disease because they help break down homocysteine, an amino acid from meat that increases the risk of vascular diseases. B vitamins also help the body produce energy to regenerate cells. They are abundant in beans, leafy green vegetables, nuts, seeds, poultry, seafood, and whole grains.

FLAVONOIDS, CAROTENOIDS, AND POLYPHENOLS

Studies correlate several antioxidant compounds found in plants with cognitive health. Of particular interest are a type of plant chemical known as polyphenols, which include the powerhouse antioxidant flavonoids. Along with carotenoids, they create the vivid colors in fruits and vegetables.

Flavonoids are very effective at protecting brain cells from damage caused by toxins and inflammation as well as improving memory and cognition. Flavonoids are found in apples, bananas, berries, citrus fruits, legumes, tea, and wine.

Carotenoids are found in bell peppers, cantaloupes, carrots, leafy green vegetables, oranges, tomatoes, watermelons, wine, and yams.

Polyphenols are found in coffee, dark chocolate, fruit and vegetables, herbs and spices, plant oils, tea, and wine.

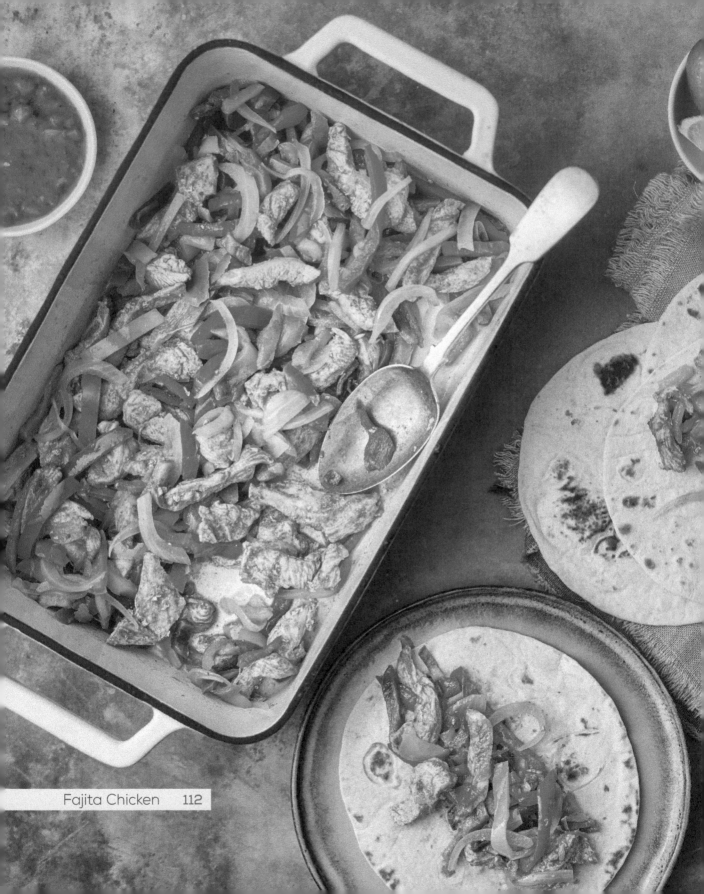

Fajita Chicken   112

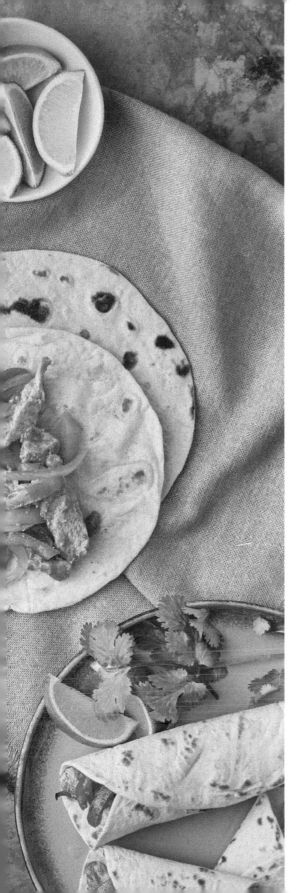

CHAPTER TWO

Foods, Nutrients, and Lifestyle

This chapter will provide a clear picture of the foods, nutrients, and lifestyle choices recommended by the MIND diet to prevent or slow the onset of cognitive decline. To obtain the most benefit, it is essential to eat MIND diet foods on a daily and weekly basis. The power players of the MIND diet include leafy greens, vegetables, berries, nuts, olive oil, whole grains, beans, seafood, and poultry.

Daily Foods

The following foods are the superstars of the MIND diet and should be eaten every day to reap the benefit of their antioxidant properties. The brain is susceptible to oxidative damage because it utilizes large quantities of oxygen to function and harmful free radicals are created naturally by these processes. Antioxidants are responsible for protecting the body from oxidative damage; experts believe they help fight the free radicals that promote chronic disease.

WHOLE GRAINS

The MIND diet does not suggest avoiding carbohydrates; rather, it suggests that you enjoy the most fiber- and nutrient-dense versions of them. Whole-grain foods are rich in B vitamins and are a moderate source of vitamin E, both of which your brain needs. If you need to avoid gluten in your diet, always check ingredient packaging for gluten-free labeling to ensure that foods were processed in a completely gluten-free facility.

Foods: Amaranth, barley, brown rice, buckwheat, bulgur, cornmeal, farro, freekeh, millet, oats, popcorn, quinoa, rye, sorghum, spelt, teff, triticale, whole wheat, wild rice

Serving recommendations: 3 servings per day of whole grains

Serving sizes: 1 slice of whole-grain bread; ½ cup of cooked brown rice, quinoa, or other cooked grain; ½ cup of cooked whole-grain pasta; ½ cup of cooked oatmeal

LEAFY GREEN VEGETABLES

Dark leafy greens are packed with vitamin C, carotenoids, and B vitamins. Greens are a powerhouse source of these vital antioxidants and are a simple delivery system that is an easy base for any salad, sandwich, or other dish.

Foods: Arugula, beet greens, bok choy, brassica, cabbage, chard, collard, dandelion, endive, kale, leeks, microgreens, mustard, radicchio, rapini, romaine, spinach, spring, turnip, watercress

Serving recommendations: 1 salad per day

Serving sizes: 1 cup of raw leafy greens or ½ cup of cooked greens

OTHER VEGETABLES

It is recommended to eat at least one additional serving of vegetables per day, aside from your leafy greens. Although one serving is recommended, you can eat as many veggies as you like, and I would encourage you to include more than one serving per day.

Foods: Artichoke, asparagus, beets, bell peppers, broccoli, Brussels sprouts, carrots, cauliflower, celery, chiles, chives, corn, cucumber, eggplant, garlic, ginger, green beans, mushrooms, okra, onions, peas, radish, sweet peppers, squash, sweet potatoes or yams, tomatoes, wax beans, zucchini

Serving recommendations: At least 1 serving per day

Serving sizes: 1 cup of raw vegetables or ½ cup of cooked vegetables

WHY VEGETABLE OILS MATTER

The MIND diet recommends vegetable oils as a source of healthy fats. Unsaturated fats help improve blood vessel function, reduce inflammation, lower blood pressure, and support cognitive functions such as neuron and synaptic transmissions and brain plasticity. You will not find a single recipe in this book that uses butter, lard, or margarine. Almost every recipe uses vegetable oils, with a preference for olive oil. In the occasional recipe, you will see canola oil or vegetable oil; these oils are a great solution when the smoke point of olive oil is too low for the cooking method or the flavor of olive oil might overwhelm the dish.

Weekly Foods

While the following foods do not have to be daily foods, it is recommended that you eat them several times per week, and it is healthy to eat them daily if you choose. Many of these foods contain fats that are beneficial to brain health as well as additional antioxidants, vitamins, and minerals that help prevent cognitive decline.

BERRIES

Berries are a surprisingly versatile fruit that are simply delicious raw, blended, cooked, canned, or preserved. Berries have been extensively studied, including by Dr. Morris, in the prevention of Alzheimer's disease and the slowing of cognitive decline. They are packed with antioxidants and other anti-inflammatory agents. All berries are wonderful, but fresh (rather than frozen) berries seem to contain the most antioxidants.

Foods: Açai berry, blackberry, blueberry, cranberry, currant, goji berry, gooseberry, raspberry, strawberry

Serving recommendations: ½ cup at least twice per week

Serving sizes: ½ cup of whole berries or ½ cup of smoothie

NUTS

Nuts are handy-dandy shelf-stable protein sources that contain brain-healthy fats and antioxidants. Nuts are fantastic fighters for brain and cardiovascular health, not to mention that they are crunchy, decadent, and tasty. Aside from snacking on nuts or having a nut butter sandwich, nuts and nut butters go beautifully in countless dishes, as you will find in this book.

Foods: Almonds, Brazil nuts, cashews, chestnuts, hazelnuts, macadamia nuts, mixed nuts, peanuts, pecans, pine nuts, pistachios, walnuts

Serving recommendations: Snack on nuts most days

Serving sizes: ¼ cup of nuts or 2 tablespoons of nut butter

SEAFOOD

A stocked MIND freezer will have frozen lean protein options at the ready. Buying protein in bulk and freezing can save you money, and most lean proteins can last up to six months in the freezer. Unless you are lucky enough to live directly on an ocean coast, the seafood you purchase is likely to be frozen. This prevents foodborne illness and does not negatively impact the nutritional value of the fish.

Foods: Anchovies, clams, cod, crab, herring, lobster, mackerel, mussels, oysters, salmon, sardines, scallops, sea bass, shrimp, squid, swordfish, trout, tuna, walleye

Serving recommendations: 1 or more servings per week

Serving size: 3 to 4 ounces of fish or seafood, about the size of a deck of cards

POULTRY

Lean poultry is an excellent source of protein. I specify "lean" because the skin, usually fried, can be a source of the saturated (bad) fat that we are trying to avoid. Baking, boiling, broiling, or grilling chicken or turkey breast with countless flavor combinations will keep your palate excited.

Foods: Skinless chicken breast, skinless turkey breast

Serving recommendations: 2 or more servings per week

Serving size: 3 to 4 ounces of chicken or turkey, about the size of a deck of cards

BEANS AND OTHER LEGUMES

Legumes, including beans, are a fiber-rich vegetarian protein source that are relied on worldwide. They also contain high amounts of B vitamins, which are important on the MIND diet. At first glance you might worry that you will be eating bean chili every night of the week, but fear not. It is easy to incorporate beans and other legumes into almost any dish, as certain recipes in this book will show.

Foods: Black beans, black-eyed peas, blue peas, cannellini beans, chickpeas (garbanzo beans) including hummus, edamame (soybeans), fava beans, great northern beans, green peas, kidney beans, lentils (any color), lima beans, mung beans, navy beans, pinto beans, split peas (green or yellow), tofu, white peas

Serving recommendations: 3 to 4 servings per week

Serving size: ½ cup of whole beans or hummus

PORTION CONTROL

Talking in cups and ounces can get confusing. Here is a visual guide to portion sizes that will help you build your plate.

FIST	**PALM**	**HANDFUL**	**THUMB**
1 cup	3–4 ounces	1 ounce	1–2 tablespoons
Leafy greens and vegetables	Seafood Poultry	Nuts Seeds	Nut butter

The following foods are not included on the official MIND diet list, but they are favorites that people often wonder about.

Fruit (beyond berries) is an excellent source for countless vitamins and minerals as well as additional antioxidants. Other fruits have not been directly proven to be effective in preventing or slowing cognitive decline, but it is completely healthy for you to enjoy all types of fruit.

Seeds, just like nuts, are fiber and protein rich and have the added benefit of healthy fats. You can enjoy seeds on the MIND diet, including chia seeds, flaxseed, pumpkin seeds, sesame seeds (and sesame products like sesame seed butter and tahini), and sunflower seeds.

Coffee, chocolate, and cocoa are antioxidant powerhouses that are not directly included in the MIND diet. It's important to read labels because many sources of chocolate are heavily processed and contain high levels of added sugar. Some recipes in this book use dark chocolate, which contains a high percentage of cacao without all the sugar and fat found in milk chocolate.

Red wine is another MIND diet choice that has brain benefits. However, drinking alcohol is a personal decision that is highly dependent on individual conditions. If you choose to consume alcohol, it's important to do so in moderation. Talk to your doctor to make sure it is safe to imbibe.

Foods to Limit

Food is to be enjoyed as well as to benefit health. Foods to limit because of saturated and trans fats do not need to be eliminated entirely; rather, they should be eaten sparingly and not regularly. Foods to be limited on the MIND diet include red meat, dairy, eggs, fried foods, sweets, and pastries.

RED MEAT

The American diet is traditionally high in red meat; beef has long been king. However, high amounts of saturated fat have been proven time and time again to be detrimental to brain and heart health.

Foods: Bacon, beef, deli meats, game meat, ground beef, ham, lamb, mutton, pork, roast beef, steak, veal, venison

Serving recommendations: No more than three servings of red meat per week; less is even better

Serving size: 3 to 5 ounces of beef or pork, about the size of a deck of cards

DAIRY, MARGARINE, AND EGGS

Dairy products, including milk, butter (even nondairy margarine), and cheese, are typically high in saturated fat. Skim or low-fat dairy products can be included in a healthy diet, but for the purpose of teaching you how to eat on the MIND diet, they will not be included in this book. It was long believed that eggs contained too much cholesterol for a healthy diet. However, current science shows that most cholesterol is produced naturally in the liver and has less to do with dietary cholesterol intake. The reason caution should be taken with eggs is because the foods that often accompany eggs (such as bacon, cheese, or pastries) are high in saturated and trans fats that are unhealthy for the heart and brain. Eggs are a part of a well-rounded diet but should be balanced with whole grains, fruits and vegetables, beans and legumes, nuts, and seeds. The recipes in this book do not include eggs.

Foods: Butter, cheese, cream cheese, creamer, eggs, frozen yogurt, half-and-half, ice cream, lactose-free milk, creamy salad dressings, margarine, pudding, reduced-fat milk, skim milk, sour cream, whipped cream, whole milk, yogurt

Serving recommendations: 1 to 2 ounces per week

Serving size: The size of your thumb for hard cheese or 2 tablespoons of crumbled cheese

FRIED FOODS AND FAST FOODS

We all have a special place for fried food and fast food in our stomachs. In addition to being indulgently delicious, they are also loaded with fat, salt, and sugar—all ingredients that do not support brain and heart health. Fried foods and fast foods should be limited as much as possible and regarded as a once-in-a-while treat.

Foods: Burgers, cheeseburgers, cheese curds, chicharrons, chicken fried steak, chiles rellenos, Chinese takeout, corn dogs, deep-fried anything, egg rolls, fast-food burritos, fast-food tacos, fish and chips, flautas, French fries, fried chicken, fried clams, fried pickles, fried shrimp, hash browns, hot dogs, hushpuppies, jalapeño poppers, mozzarella sticks, onion rings, pizza, pork rinds, taquitos, Tater Tots

Serving recommendations: Every once in a while, as little as possible

Serving size: At your discretion for a treat

SWEETS AND PASTRIES

Excess added sugar and fat do our brains and bodies no good. There is no direct evidence that sugar itself affects cognitive decline, but a healthy diet limits the intake of sweets and pastries.

Foods: Baklava, brownies, cake, candy, candy bars, cannoli, chocolate (other than dark chocolate and cocoa), cookies, croissants, cupcakes, custard, donuts, fudge, funnel cake, frozen yogurt, ice cream, pie, pudding, puff pastry, soda, sports drinks, strudel, sugary boxed cereal, tarts, tiramisu

Serving recommendations: No more than 5 servings per week

Serving size: 1 ounce of candy, 1 to 3 cookies depending on size, 1 small pastry

CAN I FOLLOW THE MIND DIET IF I DON'T EAT MEAT?

Despite the MIND diet including poultry and seafood, vegetarians and vegans can still benefit from the diet. A primary concern would be to get enough omega-3 fatty acids in your diet, but the great news is that you can do so without meat or seafood. Chia seeds, edamame, flaxseed, hemp seeds, kidney beans, seaweed, and vegetable oil are all plant sources of omega-3s. Pescatarians who won't be eating poultry will get incredible benefit from the diet and can substitute fish for any poultry portion recommended. Every recipe in this book can be easily made vegetarian or vegan by omitting the animal protein and substituting a plant protein like tofu or beans.

The MIND Diet Lifestyle

The MIND diet, much like the Mediterranean and DASH diets, isn't just about what you eat but also about making beneficial changes in your lifestyle. Exercising, getting adequate rest, reducing stress, and keeping an active mind all are important to preventing or delaying cognitive decline.

GET MOVING

A 2015 study by Jill Barnes found that along with countless other benefits, exercise helps prevent cognitive decline. Regular exercise is directly proven to reduce the prevalence and risk for high blood pressure, obesity, diabetes, and high cholesterol, all of which are linked to developing dementia. It is recommended that you get at least 150 minutes of aerobic activity at a moderate intensity per week. This includes brisk walking, jogging, running, jumping rope, body-weight exercises, swimming, biking outdoors or stationary indoors, elliptical, and dance class. Pick an activity you enjoy; there is no reason exercise should feel like a chore. If you do not like to run, you don't have to run!

SLEEP WELL

During sleep, our brain solidifies memories and flushes out toxins, among countless other imperative processes. A 2015 study published in *Current Opinions in Psychiatry* found that lack of sleep is linked to cognitive decline, obesity, diabetes, heart disease, and premature death. Make sleep a priority by waking up and going to bed around the same time each day, by avoiding caffeine and alcohol before bed, by creating a relaxing routine before bed (like reading or listening to soft music), and by avoiding TV and computer screens just before you sleep.

REDUCE STRESS AND THINK POSITIVELY

Stress increases the levels of hormones and chemicals that cause inflammation in your body, which can in turn increase your stress level, creating a cycle of chronic inflammation. The Alzheimer's Association found that a positive outlook is linked to decreased prevalence of dementia. Simple ways to reduce stress and increase positivity are to:

Get a change of scenery, like stepping outside to feel the sun or the cool breeze on your face.

Listen to a song that you enjoy or that relaxes you.

Take a short walk or perform an exercise that is comfortable for your body, like stretching or light yoga.

KEEP AN ACTIVE MIND (AND SOCIAL LIFE)

Harvard Medical School research shows that keeping an active mind is important to brain health as we age. Activities such as crossword puzzles, card games, reading, journaling, crafts, and brain games are related to decreased cognitive decline. Similarly, socialization and personal connections keep our brains active and healthy. People with close social connections are less likely to experience cognitive decline because socializing involves communication, activity, and making memories.

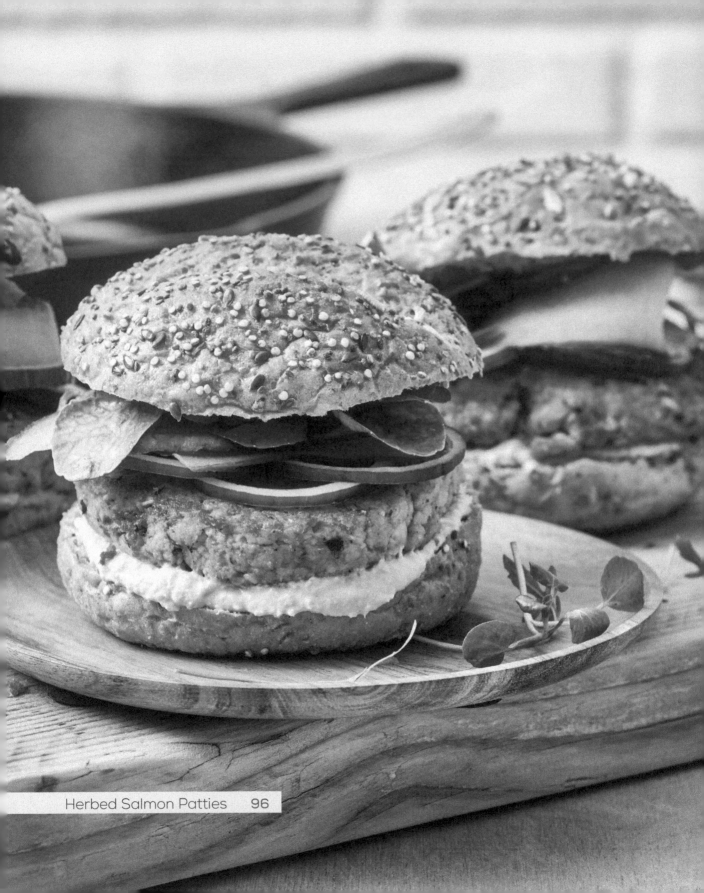

Herbed Salmon Patties   96

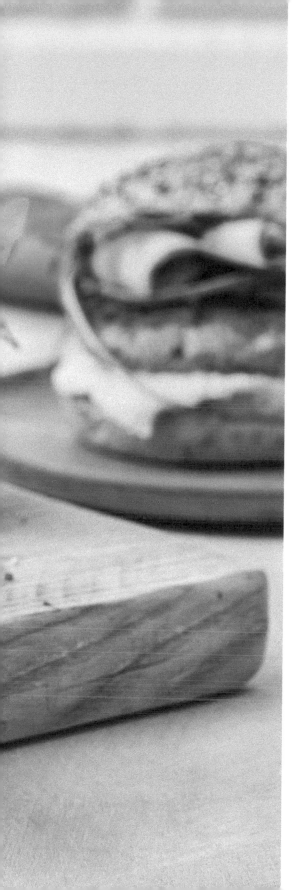

CHAPTER THREE

The 14-Day MIND Diet Meal Plan

This chapter will show you how to put the MIND diet food recommendations into practice. Creating a meal plan or "meal prepping" sounds overwhelming, but it does not have to be! Meal planning is as simple as taking a piece of scratch paper, writing down what sounds good to eat for the week, and then basing your grocery shopping list on the ingredients needed for those recipes. This is a diet meant to be enjoyed to improve your health; do not be stressed as if this were a strict fad diet and if you "fall off the wagon" you have to feel bad and quit. The MIND diet is all about encouraging you to eat healthy foods that will protect your brain.

About the Meal Plan

This 14-day meal plan is included to get you jump-started on the MIND diet with no stress. After two weeks, you will find that you can continue the diet on your own for the long haul. Because the meals are so simple and quick to prepare, I hope that starting the MIND diet is a smooth transition and that it does not have to be complicated or expensive.

The MIND diet recipes that I have developed for this book ensure that you will achieve your weekly intake of recommended foods. Most recipes have been developed to feed two people, though some will yield leftovers that you can enjoy later in the week for a quick reheated lunch. To scale a recipe up for more people, simply double or triple it, and if a recipe makes leftovers, you can cut it in half for a smaller yield. Every meal is ready in 30 minutes or less; some are even ready in under 15 minutes. You will also find that the recipes focus on pantry staples that you likely already have on hand, which means you will not have to constantly run out to the store.

I am so proud of you for diving into the meal plan and taking this next step toward better cognitive health. The recipes and weekly menus will clearly illustrate how to eat on the MIND diet. Remember, this diet should be delicious and filling rather than dull and restrictive.

If you find that you are hungry between meals, take a look at the Snacks and Sides chapter (page 49) for healthy bites to tide you over. Likewise, when your sweet tooth comes calling, enjoy any of the desserts from the Sweet Treats chapter (page 115).

Week 1 Menu

	BREAKFAST	LUNCH	DINNER
MONDAY	Tofu "Egg" Sandwich (page 38)	Berry Spring Greens (page 70)	Tuscan Bean Soup (page 72)
TUESDAY	Overnight Oatmeal (page 37)	Apple, Walnut, and Spinach Salad (page 66)	Loaded Shrimp Pasta (page 87)
WEDNESDAY	Fruit Salad (page 43)	Leftover Loaded Shrimp Pasta	Chicken Enchiladas (page 100)
THURSDAY	Rainbow Smoothie (page 34)	Leftover Tuscan Bean Soup	Herbed Salmon Patties (page 96)
FRIDAY	Overnight Oatmeal (page 37)	Leftover Chicken Enchiladas	Three-Bean Chili (page 76)
SATURDAY	Tofu "Egg" Sandwich (page 38)	Leftover Herbed Salmon Patty sandwiches	Green Chile Stew (page 74)
SUNDAY	Rainbow Smoothie (page 34)	Leftover Three-Bean Chili	Smothered Bean Burritos (page 77)

Week 1 Shopping List

PRODUCE

Apples (4)

Arugula (2 cups)

Asparagus (1 bunch)

Bananas (2)

Blueberries (2 cups)

Cabbage, shredded
(2 cups)

Carrots (4)

Celery (1 bunch)

Dill (1 bunch)

Jalapeño peppers (2)

Kale, shredded (2 cups)

Lemon (1)

Mushrooms,
sliced (1 cup)

Onions, white (2)

Raspberries (3½ cups)

Spinach (11 cups)

Spring greens (8 cups)

Strawberries (2 cups)

Tomatoes, grape or
cherry (3 cups)

Tomato, large (1)

Zucchini (1)

FROZEN FOODS

Blueberries (2 cups)

Raspberries (2 cups)

PANTRY

Basil, dried

Beans, black,
3 (15-ounce) cans, no
salt added

Beans, cannellini,
2 (15-ounce) cans, no
salt added

Beans, kidney,
1 (15-ounce) can, no
salt added

Beans, pinto,
2 (15-ounce) cans, no
salt added

Black pepper,
freshly ground

Chili powder

Chipotle chili powder

Cinnamon, ground

Cranberries, dried
(½ cup)

Cumin, ground

Flour, all-purpose

Garlic, minced,
1 (4.5-ounce) jar

Garlic powder

Green chiles, whole,
1 (27-ounce) can

Honey (4 tablespoons)

Lemon juice
(1 tablespoon plus
1 teaspoon)

Lime juice
(2 tablespoons)

Mandarin oranges,
1 (11-ounce) can

Mustard, yellow

Nonstick cooking spray

Nutmeg, ground

Nuts of choice (1 cup)

Oats, rolled (4 cups)

Olive oil

Onion powder

Oregano, dried

Panko bread crumbs
(⅓ cup)

Pasta, whole wheat
(8 ounces)

Peanut butter,
creamy (1 cup)

Peas, 1 (8.5-ounce) can

Rosemary, dried

Salmon,
2 (5-ounce) cans

Thyme, dried

Tomatoes, diced
fire-roasted, 1
(14.5-ounce) can, no
salt added

Tomatoes, petite diced,
2 (15-ounce) cans, no
salt added

Tomato paste
(2 tablespoons)

Tomato sauce,
2 (15-ounce) cans, no
salt added

Vegetable stock
(10 cups)

Vinegar, balsamic

Vinegar, white wine

Walnut pieces (1 cup)

REFRIGERATED

Chicken breast,
boneless, skinless,
precooked or canned
(8 ounces)

English muffins (8)

Nondairy milk,
unsweetened, plain
(8 cups)

Shrimp, peeled and
deveined (1 pound)

Tofu, extra-firm,
2 (14-ounce) containers

Tortillas, corn, 8 (6 inch)

Tortillas, whole
wheat (4)

Week 2 Menu

	BREAKFAST	LUNCH	DINNER
MONDAY	Veggie Pitas (page 41)	Avocado, Tomato, and Arugula Salad (page 68)	Not Your Mother's Tuna Casserole (page 95)
TUESDAY	Red Smoothie (page 35)	Leftover Not Your Mother's Tuna Casserole	Jambalaya (page 102)
WEDNESDAY	Hummus on Whole-Grain Toast (page 42)	Chickpea Sliders (page 75)	One-Pot Lentils and Rice (page 73)
THURSDAY	Veggie Pitas (page 41)	Leftover Jambalaya	Shrimp Tacos (page 92)
FRIDAY	Red Smoothie (page 35)	Leftover Shrimp Tacos	Turkey Meat Loaf (page 103)
SATURDAY	Blueberry Pancakes (page 40)	Leftover One-Pot Lentils and Rice	Dijon Salmon (page 94)
SUNDAY	Hummus on Whole-Grain Toast (page 42)	Leftover Turkey Meat Loaf sandwiches	Vegan Pesto Pasta (page 79) with left-over Dijon Salmon

Week 2 Shopping List

Make sure to check your pantry for ingredients before you head to the store! Each week you will find that you have more and more on hand in your stocked pantry.

PRODUCE

Arugula (8 cups)

Avocados (3)

Basil (2 bunches)

Beets (2)

Bell peppers, any color (2)

Bell pepper, green (1)

Blueberries (1 cup)

Carrots (2)

Celery stalks (2)

Coleslaw mix (1 cup)

Lemon (1)

Mushrooms, button (4 cups)

Onions, white (2)

Parsley (1 bunch)

Spinach (4 cups)

Tomatoes, large (2)

Tomato, small (1)

Zucchini (3)

FROZEN

Raspberries (2 cups)

Strawberries (2 cups)

PANTRY

Baking powder

Baking soda

Basil, dried

Bay leaves

Black pepper, freshly ground

Chicken stock (⅓ cup)

Chickpeas, 4 (15-ounce) cans, no salt added

Chili powder

Cinnamon, ground

Cranberry juice, 100 percent pure (2 cups)

Dijon mustard (3 tablespoons)

Garlic, minced, 1 (4.5-ounce) jar

Garlic powder

Flour, all-purpose

Honey (2 tablespoons)

Ketchup (2 tablespoons)

Lemon juice (⅔ cup)

Lentils, brown (2 cups)

Lime juice
(1 tablespoon)

Olive oil

Onion powder

Oregano, dried

Panko bread crumbs
(1½ cups)

Pasta, whole wheat,
any shape (8 ounces)

Pasta, whole wheat,
penne or rotini
(8 ounces)

Peas, 1 (8.5-ounce) can

Pine nuts
(2 tablespoons)

Rice, brown (1 cup)

Tahini (⅔ cup)

Thyme, ground

Tomato sauce,
2 (8-ounce) cans, no
salt added

Tuna, canned chunk
light, 2 (5-ounce) cans

Wild rice (1 cup)

Worcestershire sauce
(1 tablespoon)

REFRIGERATED

Bread, whole wheat
(8 slices)

Buns, whole wheat
slider (4)

Chicken breast, bone-
less and skinless
(8 ounces)

Corn tortillas, 8
(6-inch)

Nondairy milk,
unsweetened, plain
(2 cups)

Pitas, whole wheat (8)

Salmon fillets
(12 ounces)

Shrimp (1 pound)

Turkey, ground, lean
(1 pound)

Beyond the 14 Days

The recipes in this book will teach you how to integrate the MIND diet for the long term to prevent cognitive decline. After following the 14-day meal plan, you should have a strong foundation for moving forward. Feel free to get creative with the recipes—if a dish calls for tilapia and you prefer salmon, go for it! Of course, you will want to enjoy tempting foods that are not MIND diet recommended, but as you choose to eat them as a treat every once in a while, you can simply continue with your MIND diet foods at your next meal with no guilt or overcompensation required.

About the Recipes

This cookbook adheres completely to the MIND diet. This cookbook will help you prevent Alzheimer's disease and dementia with healthy, great-tasting foods. All recipes and ingredients are MIND diet–friendly and have been carefully selected to illustrate how easy it is to eat a variety of foods on the MIND diet.

MIND diet–specific foods are highlighted in each recipe for your convenience. This way, you can learn what foods fit into your diet to easily meet your meal plan requirements.

You will not find any restricted foods in any recipes. These include dairy, eggs, red meat, added salt or sugar, and trans fats. You may, of course, enjoy limited daily and weekly portions of these other foods at your own discretion.

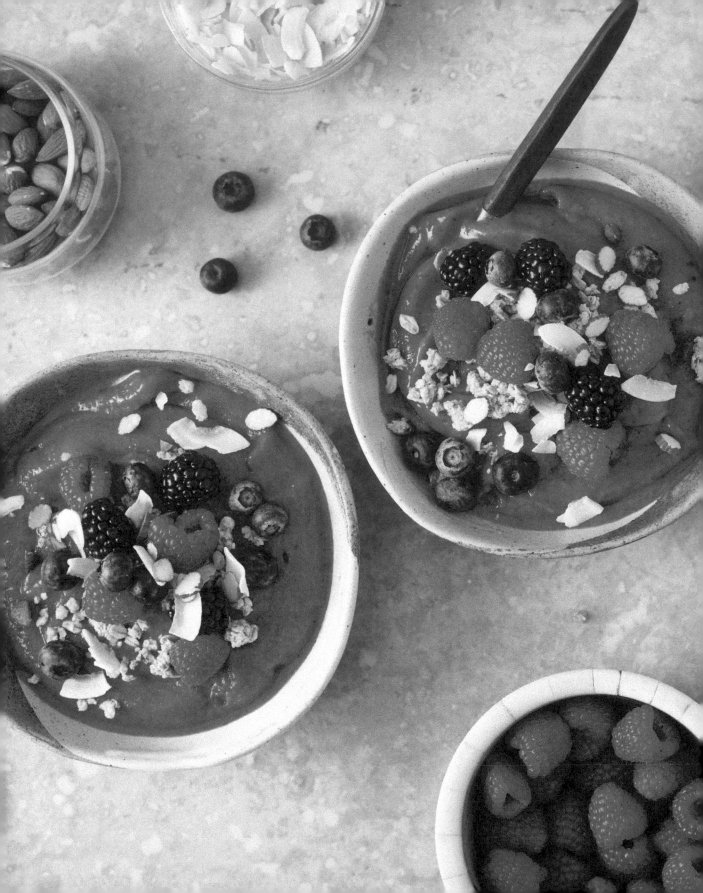

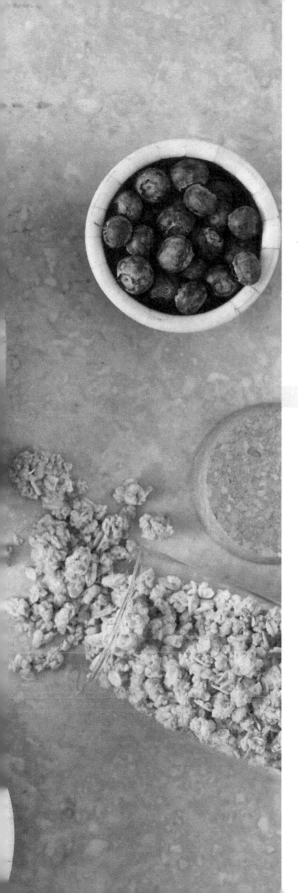

CHAPTER FOUR

Breakfasts and Smoothies

Rainbow Smoothie

Prep time: 5 minutes

SERVES 2

GLUTEN-FREE   NUT-FREE   VEGAN

Start your day with an antioxidant boost with this breakfast smoothie, featuring a rainbow of ingredients that are red, blue, green, and yellow. The banana and berries bring a bright sweetness, so you won't even notice that there is spinach in your cup!

2 cups unsweetened
plain or vanilla
nondairy milk

1 cup frozen raspberries

1 cup frozen blueberries

1 cup packed
fresh spinach

1 banana, sliced

1. Add the nondairy milk, raspberries, blueberries, spinach, and banana to a blender and process on high until smooth or on the smoothie setting for 30 to 60 seconds.

2. Add additional liquid as needed to reach your desired consistency and re-blend.

3. Serve chilled.

Ingredient tip: This is the perfect recipe to use up a banana that is overly ripe or a handful of spinach at the end of the week to reduce food waste.

Variation tip: Any blend of berries would work in this recipe. Strawberries, cranberries, blackberries, boysenberries, gooseberries, or açai berries would add nutrient-dense tanginess to this smoothie.

Per serving: Calories: 138; Total fat: 2.5g; Saturated fat: 0g; Cholesterol: 0mg; Sodium: 184mg; Carbohydrates: 28g; Fiber: 6.5g; Sugar: 15g; Protein: 2g

Red Smoothie

Prep time: 5 minutes

SERVES 2

GLUTEN-FREE **NUT-FREE** VEGAN

This bold red smoothie is so beautiful you will be racing to take the first sip. Anthocyanins are the antioxidants that give foods like beets their red color, and they are MIND diet superstars. You can use a fresh beet, or to skip peeling and dicing, you can use prepackaged beets from the refrigerated produce section of the grocery store.

1 red beet, peeled and diced

1 cup frozen strawberries

1 cup frozen raspberries

1 cup 100 percent cranberry juice

1 cup water

1. Add the beet, strawberries, raspberries, cranberry juice, and water to a blender and process on high until smooth or on the smoothie setting for 30 to 60 seconds.

2. Add additional liquid as needed to reach your desired consistency and re-blend.

3. Serve chilled.

Cooking tip: Be sure to wash your cutting board and countertops right after preparing the beets. Beet juice is a vibrant red that stains almost instantly!

Per serving: Calories: 120; Total fat: 0g; Saturated fat: 0g; Cholesterol: 0mg; Sodium: 37mg; Carbohydrates: 30g; Fiber: 3.5g; Sugar: 23g; Protein: 2g

Smoothie Bowl

Prep time: 5 minutes

SERVES 2

GLUTEN-FREE   NUT-FREE   VEGAN

A smoothie bowl is a fun way to start your day; it is like eating a sundae for breakfast! Take an extra minute to decorate your smoothie bowl with tasty toppings to make a creative masterpiece and to incorporate a variety of textures.

FOR THE SMOOTHIE

2 frozen bananas

2 cups frozen
   strawberries

1 cup frozen blackberries

¼ cup cold water

**FOR TOPPINGS
(ALL OPTIONAL)**

Sliced fresh fruit

Chopped almonds,
   walnuts, or pecans

Dried or toasted coconut

Grape-Nuts cereal

Cornflakes

Dark chocolate chips

Granola

Drizzle nut butter

TO MAKE THE SMOOTHIE

1. Add the bananas, strawberries, blackberries, and water to a blender and process on high or on the smoothie setting for 30 to 60 seconds.

2. Divide the smoothie into two bowls.

TO MAKE THE SMOOTHIE BOWLS

3. Decorate the bowls with toppings (if using) and serve.

Cooking tip: A smoothie bowl has an almost sorbet-like texture and is thicker and more luscious than a smoothie. To make any smoothie into a smoothie bowl, simply add less liquid.

Ingredient tip: Whenever you have bananas about to turn, peel them and pop them in a freezer-safe bag or container for your next smoothie.

Per serving (without toppings): Calories: 185; Total fat: 0.5g; Saturated fat: 0g; Cholesterol: 0mg; Sodium: 5mg; Carbohydrates: 47g; Fiber: 6.5g; Sugar: 27g; Protein: 3g

Overnight Oatmeal

Prep time: 10 minutes, plus refrigerating overnight
SERVES 4
CONTAINS NUTS GLUTEN-FREE ONE-POT **VEGETARIAN**

Overnight oats require no cooking because the oats absorb the liquid overnight, softening them and infusing them with the flavors you have included. You can make a large batch of overnight oatmeal to last you the entire week in just 10 minutes!

2 cups unsweetened plain or vanilla nondairy milk

2 cups rolled oats

½ cup creamy or crunchy nut butter

1 tablespoon honey or maple syrup

¾ cup fresh raspberries

1. In a large bowl or airtight container, combine the nondairy milk, oats, nut butter, and honey. Stir well.

2. Top the oats with the raspberries and seal the container with plastic wrap or an airtight lid.

3. Place in the refrigerator overnight to soak and enjoy in the morning. Overnight oats are traditionally served chilled. Store leftovers in an airtight container in the refrigerator for 3 to 4 days.

Variation tip: You can flavor your overnight oats however you like. If there is a sweet breakfast you love, I bet you can translate it into overnight oats. For example, I replicate my favorite, cinnamon rolls, by adding cinnamon, honey, a pinch of salt, and sliced apples to my overnight oats.

Per serving: Calories: 400; Total fat: 22g; Saturated fat: 2.5g; Cholesterol: 0mg; Sodium: 158mg; Carbohydrates: 43g; Fiber: 11g; Sugar: 9g; Protein: 13g

Tofu "Egg" Sandwich

Prep time: 20 minutes   Cook time: 10 minutes

SERVES 4

NUT-FREE   VEGAN

Tofu, or soybean curd, is an excellent source of vegetable-based protein and strong antioxidants. Tofu does not have a robust flavor on its own, making it a great blank canvas for recipes like this one where it is the star of this simple, tasty sandwich.

14 ounces extra-firm tofu

2 teaspoons olive oil

½ teaspoon jarred minced garlic

4 whole wheat English muffins or 8 slices of whole wheat bread

Yellow mustard

Freshly ground black pepper

1 cup grape or cherry tomatoes, quartered

1 cup arugula or spinach

1. Line a plate with a thick stack of paper towels and set aside.

2. Remove the tofu block from the package, drain the water, and slice the block horizontally into 4 thin and wide slices.

3. Place the slices in a single layer on the paper towels, add additional paper towels on top of the tofu, and place a cutting board on top of the paper towels. Weigh the cutting board down with a heavy book, a pot, or several cans. Leave the tofu to be pressed for at least 15 minutes.

4. In a large pan or skillet, heat the olive oil and garlic over medium heat until shimmering; then add the slices of tofu.

5. Cook the tofu for 5 minutes, flip the tofu over, and cook for another 5 minutes. The tofu will begin to lightly brown.

6. While the tofu is cooking, toast the English muffins.

7. Build each sandwich starting with the bottom of an English muffin, a swirl of mustard, a slice of tofu, a sprinkle of black pepper, tomatoes, and arugula. Add the English muffin top to close the sandwich and serve.

Ingredient tip: Pressing the tofu takes time but is worth the effort. Watery tofu cooks down to be overly soft, whereas pressed tofu retains its firmness and can absorb more flavor from your seasonings.

Per serving: Calories: 258; Total fat: 8.5g; Saturated fat: 1g; Cholesterol: 0mg; Sodium: 292mg; Carbohydrates: 33g; Fiber: 2g; Sugar: 3g; Protein: 16g

Blueberry Pancakes

Prep time: 10 minutes   Cook time: 20 minutes

SERVES 4

NUT-FREE VEGETARIAN

These seven-ingredient pancakes are sure to become a household favorite. They are completely customizable, from the type of flour you prefer to the fruit or flavors you'd like to include.

Nonstick cooking spray

2 cups all-purpose flour

1½ tablespoons baking powder

2 teaspoons ground cinnamon

2 cups unsweetened plain or vanilla nondairy milk

1 cup fresh blueberries (more if you like)

¼ cup olive oil

1 tablespoon honey

1. Preheat a large nonstick pan or a pan lightly sprayed with cooking oil over medium heat.

2. In a large bowl, whisk together the flour, baking powder, and cinnamon. Add the nondairy milk, blueberries, olive oil, and honey and mix well.

3. Pour the batter into the pan to form the pancakes (¼ cup at a time for small pancakes or ½ cup at a time for large pancakes), as many as you can fit in your pan. Cook the batter for 3 minutes, until bubbles appear on the surface; then carefully flip the pancakes and cook for 2 minutes. The pancakes will be a light golden brown.

4. Repeat step 3 until all the batter is cooked.

5. Serve warm and enjoy the blueberry goodness.

Did you know? Cooking blueberries increases the levels of certain antioxidants they contain. Fresh, frozen, and cooked blueberries are all great options on the MIND diet.

Per serving: Calories: 411; Total fat: 16g; Saturated fat: 2g; Cholesterol: 0mg; Sodium: 87mg; Carbohydrates: 61g; Fiber: 4g; Sugar: 8.5g; Protein: 7g

Veggie Pitas

Prep time: 5 minutes   Cook time: 15 minutes
SERVES 4
NUT-FREE VEGAN

Pita bread is a yeast-leavened wheat bread that originated in the Mediterranean and Middle Eastern regions. The baking process creates an air pocket inside the bread, perfect for filling with tasty ingredients to create a mess-free handheld sandwich that is ideal for mornings when you're rushing out the door.

1 tablespoon olive oil

1 bell pepper, any color, cut into strips

½ cup sliced mushrooms

1 teaspoon dried basil

1 teaspoon dried oregano

1 zucchini, cut into half-moons

4 whole wheat pitas

1 cup fresh spinach

1. In a large pan, heat the olive oil over medium heat until shimmering.

2. Add the bell pepper, mushrooms, basil, and oregano and cook for 10 to 15 minutes, or until tender.

3. Add the zucchini during the last 5 minutes of cooking to prevent it from getting overly soft.

4. Fill each pita with ¼ cup of spinach and ¼ of the veggie mixture and serve.

Variation tip: This breakfast is a great way to use up veggies left over from the week's meals. Any vegetables will work great in this pita pocket breakfast.

Per serving: Calories: 190; Total fat: 5g; Saturated fat: 0.5g; Cholesterol: 0mg; Sodium: 246mg; Carbohydrates: 31g; Fiber: 5.5g; Sugar: 4g; Protein: 9g

Hummus on Whole-Grain Toast

Prep time: 10 minutes   Cook time: 20 minutes

SERVES 4

NUT-FREE   VEGAN

Chickpeas are a plant-based protein powerhouse. Rich in fiber, manganese, copper, and folate, these marble-size beans are a versatile pantry staple. The rich, deep flavor of this hummus is provided by tahini (sesame seed butter) and olive oil, both of which have brain-friendly anti-inflammatory properties.

1 (15-ounce) can no-salt-added chickpeas, drained and rinsed

2 cups water

¼ teaspoon baking soda

4 slices whole wheat bread

⅓ cup tahini

2 tablespoons lemon juice

2 tablespoons ice-cold water

1 tablespoon olive oil

1 teaspoon jarred minced garlic

1. In a medium saucepan, cover the chickpeas with 2 cups of water and add the baking soda.

2. Boil the chickpeas for 20 minutes, until the skins are falling off.

3. While the chickpeas are cooking, toast the bread and set aside.

4. Drain and rinse the chickpeas.

5. Add the chickpeas, tahini, lemon juice, ice-cold water, olive oil, and garlic to a blender and process for 2 to 3 minutes, until creamy and smooth.

6. Serve each piece of toast with a thick schmear of hummus.

Substitution tip: Store-bought hummus is convenient and available in a wide variety of flavors. Just be sure to check the label, as some brands are high in sodium.

Per serving: Calories: 376; Total fat: 17g; Saturated fat: 2g; Cholesterol: 0mg; Sodium: 245mg; Carbohydrates: 43g; Fiber: 8g; Sugar: 6g; Protein: 12g

Fruit Salad

Prep time: 15 minutes

SERVES 4

GLUTEN-FREE   NUT-FREE   ONE-POT   **VEGETARIAN**

Fruit salad, often considered a side dish, makes a yummy breakfast or even a fresh and easy dessert. It is an antioxidant-rich way to start your day with a medley of textures and flavors. Feel free to add chopped nuts for a crunchy protein boost.

1 cup fresh strawberries, quartered

1 cup fresh blueberries

1 cup fresh raspberries

2 small apples, diced

1 (11-ounce) can mandarin oranges in 100 percent juice, drained

2 tablespoons lime juice

2 tablespoons honey

1 teaspoon dried basil

1. In a large bowl, combine the strawberries, blueberries, raspberries, apples, and mandarin oranges.

2. In a small bowl, whisk together the lime juice, honey, and basil.

3. Mix the dressing into the fruit salad and serve.

Variation tip: Any of your favorite fruits work in this fruit salad. The recipe is merely a shell, offering endless variety to your menu.

Per serving: Calories: 177; Total fat: 0.5g; Saturated fat: 0g; Cholesterol: 0mg; Sodium: 3mg; Carbohydrates: 45g; Fiber: 7g; Sugar: 34g; Protein: 2g

Sweet Potato Hash

Prep time: 10 minutes   Cook time: 20 minutes

SERVES 4

GLUTEN-FREE **NUT-FREE** ONE-POT **VEGAN**

Sweet potatoes are not just for brown sugar and marshmallows. Here they amp up the flavor and brain health benefits to diner-style hash. The chickpeas make the dish filling and satisfying; you won't even miss the eggs!

2 tablespoons olive oil

2 large sweet potatoes, cut into ½-inch cubes

1 (15-ounce) can no-salt-added chickpeas, drained

1 red bell pepper, diced

1 cup chopped kale

2 tablespoons tahini

1 tablespoon lemon juice

Freshly ground black pepper

1 large avocado, sliced

1. In a large and deep pan, heat the olive oil over medium heat until shimmering.

2. Add the sweet potatoes, chickpeas, bell pepper, and kale and cook for 15 to 20 minutes, stirring occasionally, until the sweet potatoes are fork-tender.

3. Take the pan off the heat, and add the tahini, lemon juice, and pepper to taste. Mix until the vegetables are evenly coated.

4. Serve each plate with sliced avocado.

Did you know? Sweet potatoes are often misnamed as yams, but they are different species entirely. Sweet potatoes are rich in the antioxidant beta-carotene and vitamins A, B_6, and C. They are a great substitute for white potatoes to boost antioxidants in your diet.

Per serving: Calories: 334; Total fat: 18g; Saturated fat: 2g; Cholesterol: 0mg; Sodium: 53mg; Carbohydrates: 38g; Fiber: 11g; Sugar: 6g; Protein: 9g

Chilaquiles

Prep time: 10 minutes   Cook time: 20 minutes
SERVES 4
GLUTEN-FREE NUT-FREE VEGAN

Chilaquiles are a traditional Mexican dish consisting of fried corn tortillas softened with salsa and served with beans, meat, eggs, and cheese. These MIND diet–friendly veggie chilaquiles don't skimp on the flavor, just the saturated fat!

5 corn tortillas

1 (15-ounce) can no-salt-added black beans, drained

1 (14.5-ounce) can no-salt-added diced fire-roasted tomatoes

1 cup canned corn, drained

1 cup low-sodium vegetable broth

2 teaspoons ground cumin

¼ cup tahini

2 tablespoons cold water

1 tablespoon hot sauce

1 large avocado, diced

1. In a large pan, heat the corn tortillas in small batches over high heat until they become slightly crisp, bubbling, and browned. Cut into quarters and set aside.

2. In a large and deep pan or pot, combine the black beans, tomatoes and their juices, corn, vegetable broth, and cumin. Cook over medium-high heat for 10 minutes, until the beans are tender and most of the liquid has evaporated.

3. While the vegetables cook, in a small bowl, whisk together the tahini, water, and hot sauce.

4. Fold the corn tortilla quarters into the black bean mixture and cook together for 5 minutes until the tortillas begin to soften.

5. Serve the chilaquiles with diced avocado and a drizzle of the tahini sauce.

Substitution tip: You can use tortilla chips in place of making your own, but try to find an option that is low in sodium.

Per serving: Calories: 337; Total fat: 15g; Saturated fat: 2g; Cholesterol: 0mg; Sodium: 181mg; Carbohydrates: 41g; Fiber: 11g; Sugar: 5.5g; Protein: 12g

Quinoa Porridge

Prep time: 10 minutes   Cook time: 15 minutes

SERVES 4

CONTAINS NUTS GLUTEN-FREE ONE-POT VEGETARIAN

This quinoa porridge is an updated version of classic breakfast oatmeal. The texture of the quinoa, a protein-rich whole grain, pairs wonderfully with mouthwatering toppings of fresh fruit and almonds. Make a large batch to last you through the week.

2 cups unsweetened plain or vanilla nondairy milk

1 cup quinoa

1 tablespoon honey or maple syrup

½ teaspoon ground cinnamon

1 cup fresh fruit (like raspberries, strawberries, or peaches)

¼ cup sliced almonds

1. In a medium pot, combine the nondairy milk, quinoa, honey, and cinnamon. Bring to a simmer over medium-high heat. Reduce the heat to low, cover, and cook for 15 minutes, until the liquid has been mostly absorbed.

2. Let the porridge sit for 5 minutes.

3. Serve each bowl of porridge with ¼ cup of fresh fruit and 1 tablespoon of sliced almonds.

Cooking tip: Before cooking, rinse the quinoa with cold water to wash away any debris.

Per serving: Calories: 237; Total fat: 7g; Saturated fat: 0.5g; Cholesterol: 0mg; Sodium: 88mg; Carbohydrates: 37g; Fiber: 6.5g; Sugar: 7g; Protein: 8g

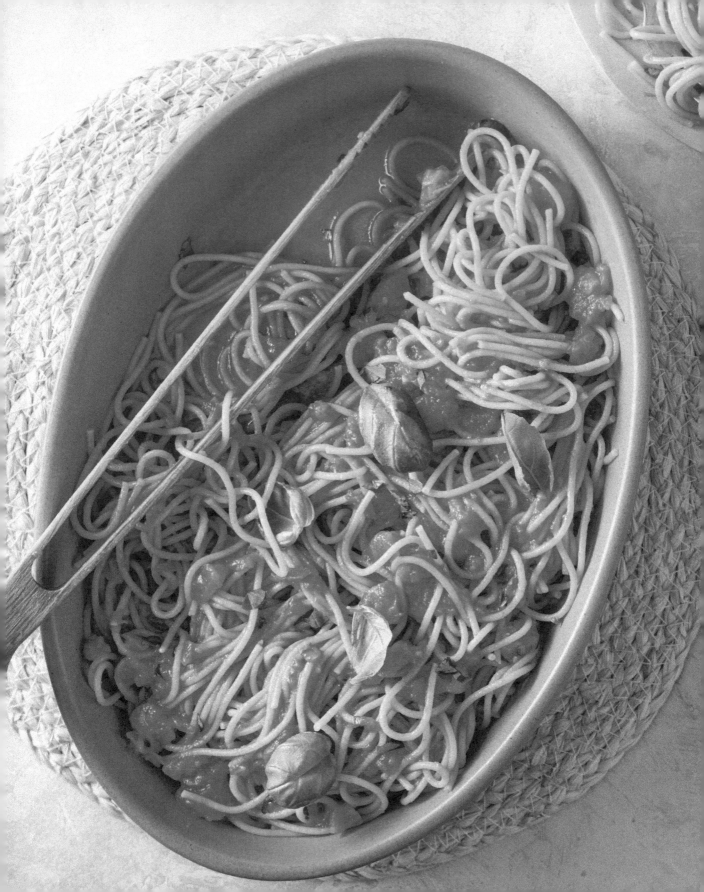

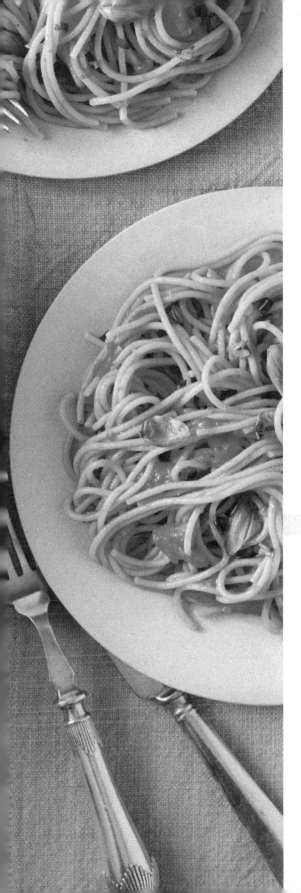

"Ranch" Popcorn

Prep time: 5 minutes   Cook time: 5 minutes

SERVES 4

GLUTEN-FREE   NUT-FREE   VEGAN

Popcorn isn't just for the movies anymore! Gone are the days of butter-loaded, salt-laden popcorn in front of a screen. Enjoy snacking on popcorn as a whole-grain, healthy MIND diet staple when you dress it up with this herb combination that is sure to delight.

2 tablespoons olive oil

½ cup popcorn kernels

½ teaspoon dried
dill weed

½ teaspoon dried chives

½ teaspoon garlic powder

½ teaspoon onion powder

1. In a large stockpot, heat the olive oil over medium heat until shimmering.

2. Add the popcorn kernels and cover the pot.

3. The kernels will pop for 4 to 5 minutes. Listen closely and when the popping slows to only every few seconds, the popcorn is done.

4. Transfer the popcorn to a large bowl. While the popcorn is hot, toss it with the dill, chives, garlic powder, and onion powder for 10 seconds and serve.

Variation tip: Popcorn is a great canvas to flavor any way you like, keeping the possibilities endless. Try cinnamon sugar or a combination of chili powder and lime zest!

Per serving: Calories: 141; Total fat: 8g; Saturated fat: 1g; Cholesterol: 0mg; Sodium: 7mg; Carbohydrates: 20g; Fiber: 4g; Sugar: 0g; Protein: 3g

Cinnamon Roasted Nuts

Prep time: 15 minutes   Cook time: 10 minutes
SERVES 4
CONTAINS NUTS GLUTEN-FREE VEGETARIAN

When I think of cinnamon roasted nuts, I am immediately taken to the ballpark, as they are always a must-have for any ball game. Even better is that you can make the crunchy, sweet treat full of protein, healthy fats, and antioxidants in your own home. Enjoy them on their own or use them to add some crunch to oatmeal or Quinoa Porridge (page 46).

½ cup raw almonds
½ cup raw cashews
½ cup raw walnuts
½ cup raw pecans
1 tablespoon olive oil
1 tablespoon honey
2 teaspoons ground
  cinnamon

1. Preheat the oven to 350°F. Line a baking sheet with parchment paper and set aside.

2. In a large bowl, toss the nuts in the olive oil, honey, and cinnamon until evenly coated.

3. On the prepared baking sheet, spread the nuts in a single layer.

4. Roast the nuts for 10 minutes, until the honey starts to caramelize.

5. Let the nuts cool for 10 minutes before serving.

Variation tip: You can use any blend of nuts you like to make these roasted nuts your new favorite!

Per serving: Calories: 388; Total fat: 35g; Saturated fat: 3.5g; Cholesterol: 0mg; Sodium: 3mg; Carbohydrates: 14g; Fiber: 5.5g; Sugar: 4g; Protein: 9g

Guacamole with Corn Chips

Prep time: 15 minutes   Cook time: 10 minutes

SERVES 4

GLUTEN-FREE   NUT-FREE   VEGAN

This snack is the best of all worlds, loaded with whole grains, fruits, vegetables, fiber, healthy fat, vitamins, minerals, and antioxidants. Corn is a whole grain, and corn tortillas are simply made of ground corn and water, with no added salt or fat. Guacamole is as healthy as it is delicious because avocados are rich in omega-3 fatty acids and tomatoes are full of antioxidants.

FOR THE CORN CHIPS

16 corn tortillas

2 tablespoons olive oil

½ tablespoon paprika

FOR THE GUACAMOLE

3 medium
   avocados, diced

1 small red onion,
   finely diced

½ cup diced tomatoes,
   fresh or canned

1 jalapeño, finely diced

1 lime, halved

1 tablespoon jarred
   minced garlic

¼ teaspoon ground
   cayenne pepper

TO MAKE THE CORN CHIPS

1. Preheat the oven to 350°F. Line a baking sheet with parchment paper and set aside.

2. While the oven is heating, brush the corn tortillas with olive oil and sprinkle evenly with paprika. Cut the seasoned tortillas into quarters. On the prepared baking sheet, arrange the tortilla pieces into a single layer or as close to a single layer as your baking sheet will allow.

3. Bake the tortilla pieces for 10 minutes until they begin to brown. The chips may feel soft but will crisp further as they cool.

TO MAKE THE GUACAMOLE

4. While the chips are cooking, in a medium bowl, mash the avocados until they are mostly smooth. Add the onion, tomatoes, jalapeño, juice of half a lime, garlic, and cayenne pepper and mix well.

5. When the chips are done baking, squeeze the juice from the remaining lime half over the chips. Allow 10 minutes to cool.

6. Serve the guacamole and corn chips together as a delicious light snack.

Ingredient tip: When shopping for corn tortillas, touch is a must to choose a good package. Lightly bend the package to see if the tortillas are fresh. If the tortillas appear to be separate, do not stick together, and are pliable, they are fresh. Corn tortillas made by small or family-run tortillerias tend to be fresher than tortillas that are mass-produced.

Per serving: Calories: 391; Total fat: 25g; Saturated fat: 3g, Cholesterol: 0mg; Sodium: 11mg; Carbohydrates: 42g; Fiber: 10g; Sugar: 2g; Protein: 7g

White Bean Hummus

Prep time: 10 minutes   Cook time: 20 minutes

SERVES 4

GLUTEN-FREE NUT-FREE VEGAN

Use canned cannellini beans or great northern beans to quickly whip up this creamy white bean hummus in the blender. Tahini and olive oil are both rich in antioxidants and have anti-inflammatory properties, making hummus a healthy way to snack. Serve the hummus on sandwiches and wraps or as a dip for vegetables, crackers, or pita chips.

1 (15-ounce) can no-salt-added white beans, like cannellini or great northern, drained and rinsed

2 cups water

⅓ cup tahini

2 tablespoons ice-cold water

2 tablespoons lemon juice

1 teaspoon jarred minced garlic

⅛ teaspoon freshly ground black pepper

1 tablespoon olive oil

1. In a medium saucepan, cover the beans with 2 cups of water and boil for 20 minutes, until very tender.

2. Drain the water and add the beans to a blender along with the tahini, ice-cold water, lemon juice, garlic, and pepper and blend for 2 to 3 minutes, until creamy and smooth.

3. Serve in a bowl with the olive oil drizzled on top.

Did you know? Hummus is traditionally made with chickpeas, but you can make it with any bean or legume that you have on hand! No matter what you choose, you will be getting protein, fiber, and brain-boosting benefits.

Per serving: Calories: 238; Total fat: 14g; Saturated fat: 2g; Cholesterol: 0mg; Sodium: 12mg; Carbohydrates: 20g; Fiber: 6g; Sugar: 1g; Protein: 9g

Peanut Butter Balls

Prep time: 30 minutes
MAKES 16 BITES
CONTAINS NUTS GLUTEN-FREE VEGETARIAN

Peanuts are a plant-based protein source rich in unsaturated fat and omega-6 fatty acids. They also contain other vitamins and minerals, including the antioxidant vitamin E. These delicious bites are a rich treat and feel much more indulgent and grown-up than your average peanut butter sandwich.

1 cup rolled oats
¾ cup creamy
  peanut butter
1 tablespoon honey
1 teaspoon vanilla extract
¼ teaspoon ground
  cinnamon
½ cup finely
  crushed peanuts

1. In a large bowl, combine the oats, peanut butter, honey, vanilla, and cinnamon until well mixed.

2. On a plate, lay out the crushed peanuts.

3. Taking 2 tablespoons of the mixture at a time, roll the dough into balls. Roll each ball in the crushed peanuts and set aside on a plate.

4. Freeze the bites for 20 minutes.

5. Store in an airtight container in the refrigerator.

Substitution tip: Make this recipe nut-free by substituting sunflower seed butter for the peanut butter and chopped sunflower seeds for the crushed peanuts.

Per serving (1 peanut butter ball): Calories: 122; Total fat: 9g; Saturated fat: 1.5g; Cholesterol: 0mg; Sodium: 52mg; Carbohydrates: 8g; Fiber: 1.5g; Sugar: 2.5g; Protein: 5g

Mushroom Caps

Prep time: 15 minutes   Cook time: 15 minutes
SERVES 4
CONTAINS NUTS VEGAN

Mushrooms are tender, earthy flavor bombs rich in B vitamins, minerals from the soil, and powerful antioxidants. They are often diced up and concealed in dishes, but this side dish makes them the star by stuffing them with a walnut-and-bread-crumb filling.

9 medium white button mushrooms

½ cup bread crumbs or panko bread crumbs

½ cup finely chopped walnuts or pecans

2 tablespoons olive oil

½ teaspoon jarred minced garlic

½ tablespoon dried oregano

1. Preheat the oven to 400°F. Line a baking sheet with parchment paper and set aside.

2. Prepare the mushrooms by slicing off the stems or snapping them from the caps. Dice the stems and place them in a bowl.

3. Gently brush the dirt from the mushroom caps with a paper towel; if you need to rinse them with water, do so briefly so as not to make the mushrooms soggy. Set the mushroom caps on the prepared baking sheet.

4. In the bowl, combine the bread crumbs, walnuts, olive oil, garlic, and oregano with the diced mushroom stems. Mix well.

5. Spoon the filling into the mushroom caps, about 2 tablespoons per mushroom cap.

6. Bake the mushroom caps uncovered for 15 minutes or until softened. Serve warm.

Did you know? The antioxidants found in mushrooms have been found to specifically fight age-related diseases including Alzheimer's disease.

Per serving: Calories: 213; Total fat: 17g; Saturated fat: 2g; Cholesterol: 0mg; Sodium: 78mg; Carbohydrates: 12g; Fiber: 2g; Sugar: 2g; Protein: 5g

Roasted Vegetables

Prep time: 10 minutes   Cook time: 20 minutes
SERVES 4
GLUTEN-FREE NUT-FREE VEGAN

This recipe calls for specific vegetables, but the more veggies the merrier! Feel free to toss in whatever veggies you have on hand. When we think root vegetables, potatoes get a lot of attention, but other root veggies like parsnips, turnips, yams, beets, rutabaga, and carrots are also delicious roasted and bring some nice variety to the table.

1 zucchini, cut into 1-inch-thick slices

1 small sweet potato, cut into ½-inch cubes

1 cup grape or cherry tomatoes

1 yellow bell pepper, cut into strips

3 tablespoons olive oil

1 tablespoon dried thyme

1 tablespoon dried rosemary

Salt

1. Preheat the oven to 400°F. Line a baking sheet with parchment paper.

2. On the prepared baking sheet, spread the zucchini, sweet potato, tomatoes, and bell pepper in a single layer.

3. Drizzle the vegetables with the oil and sprinkle with the thyme, rosemary, and salt to taste.

4. Bake for 20 minutes, until the edges of the vegetables are crispy, but watch carefully to prevent burning.

Cooking tip: If you have leftover cooked vegetables from the week, you can spray them with cooking oil and pop them in the oven to crisp them back up for a roasted vegetable feast.

Per serving: Calories: 140; Total fat: 11g; Saturated fat: 1.5g; Cholesterol: 0mg; Sodium: 373mg; Carbohydrates: 13g; Fiber: 2.5g; Sugar: 4g; Protein: 2g

Rice Pilaf

Prep time: 5 minutes   Cook time: 25 minutes

SERVES 4

NUT-FREE ONE-POT

When I think of rice pilaf, I think of an expensive, mouthwatering dish from an upscale restaurant or a salt-laden dish from a cardboard box. This rice pilaf is neither of these things because it is made from our MIND diet pantry favorites, is ready in 30 minutes, and is low in sodium.

2 tablespoons olive oil

½ cup whole wheat
　spaghetti broken into
　½-inch pieces

1¾ cups low-sodium
　chicken stock

1 cup frozen peas and
　carrots mix

¾ cup brown rice

1 tablespoon
　dried parsley

1 tablespoon dried basil

1. In a large pot, heat the olive oil over medium heat until shimmering. Toast the broken spaghetti for up to 5 minutes, until fragrant and browning.

2. Add the chicken stock, peas and carrots, rice, parsley, and basil and bring to a boil over high heat.

3. Reduce the heat to low, cover the pot, and cook for 20 minutes, or until the rice is cooked through and can be fluffed with a fork.

Variation tip: Feel free to substitute any vegetables of your choosing into this pilaf. It is a great recipe to use up scraps at the end of the week.

Per serving: Calories: 301; Total fat: 8.5g; Saturated fat: 1.5g; Cholesterol: 2mg; Sodium: 51mg; Carbohydrates: 48g; Fiber: 5g; Sugar: 2g; Protein: 10g

58   THE 30-MINUTE MIND DIET COOKBOOK

Caprese-Inspired Pasta

Prep time: 5 minutes   Cook time: 15 minutes
SERVES 4
NUT-FREE VEGAN

Caprese is a fresh Italian salad that contains mozzarella, tomato, basil, olive oil, and salt. This warm pasta dish shares the delicious flavors of caprese salad minus the cheese, making it MIND diet–friendly.

12 ounces medium-size whole wheat pasta noodles

1 (14.5-ounce) can no-salt-added diced tomatoes, drained

3 tablespoons olive oil

2 tablespoons chopped fresh basil

2 teaspoons balsamic vinegar (optional)

1 teaspoon garlic powder

1. Bring a large pot of water to a boil over high heat. Add the pasta and boil for 8 to 12 minutes, until tender.

2. While the pasta is cooking, in a large bowl, combine the tomatoes, olive oil, basil, balsamic vinegar (if using), and garlic powder.

3. Drain the pasta and transfer it to the large bowl. Mix the ingredients together and serve warm.

Substitution tip: Make this recipe gluten-free by substituting your favorite gluten-free pasta.

Per serving: Calories: 464; Total fat: 14g; Saturated fat: 2g; Cholesterol: 0mg; Sodium: 23mg; Carbohydrates: 75g; Fiber: 11g; Sugar: 4.5g; Protein: 15g

Smashed Red Potatoes

Prep time: 5 minutes   Cook time: 30 minutes

SERVES 4

GLUTEN-FREE   NUT-FREE   VEGAN

Are you ready for the most delicious, unbelievably simple two-ingredient recipe? These smashed red potatoes are crispy on the outside and creamy on the inside. They are the perfect companion to just about any meal.

8 small to medium red potatoes

2 tablespoons olive oil

1. Preheat the oven to 450°F. Line a baking sheet with aluminum foil and set aside.

2. On a microwave-safe plate, microwave the potatoes for 5 to 10 minutes, until fork-tender.

3. Carefully, using a hot pad or dish towel to protect your hand, smash each potato with the heel of your hand until all the potatoes are flattened.

4. Place the smashed potatoes on the prepared baking sheet and drizzle with the olive oil. Bake for 20 minutes, until crispy and browned.

Cooking tip: You can boil the potatoes instead of microwaving if you prefer, but it takes a bit longer.

Per serving: Calories: 328; Total fat: 7g; Saturated fat: 1g; Cholesterol: 0mg; Sodium: 69mg; Carbohydrates: 61g; Fiber: 6.5g; Sugar: 5g; Protein: 7g

Red Pepper Squash

Prep time: 5 minutes   Cook time: 30 minutes

SERVES 4

GLUTEN-FREE   NUT-FREE   VEGAN

This stuffed squash recipe is quite literally stuffed with antioxidants. In a fun play on classic stuffed peppers, in this recipe the peppers make up the filling, and beautiful roasted butternut squash provides the brain-friendly vessel.

1 butternut squash,
   halved and seeded

2 tablespoons olive oil

Salt

8 ounces
   mushrooms, sliced

1 red bell pepper, diced

1 tablespoon lemon juice

½ tablespoon
   dried oregano

½ tablespoon dried basil

1. Preheat the oven to 400°F. Line a baking sheet with foil.

2. Rub the inside of the squash halves with olive oil, sprinkle with salt to taste, and place on the prepared baking sheet cut-side up.

3. In a small bowl, combine the mushrooms, bell pepper, lemon juice, oregano, and basil. Spoon half of the mixture into each half of the butternut squash.

4. Roast the squash for 30 minutes, until tender.

5. To enjoy, scoop each bite from the center until nothing remains but the skin, which you can discard.

Per serving: Calories: 191; Total fat: 7.5g; Saturated fat: 1g; Cholesterol: 0mg; Sodium: 305mg; Carbohydrates: 32g; Fiber: 6g; Sugar: 7.5g; Protein: 5g

Roasted Brussels Sprouts

Prep time: 5 minutes   Cook time: 30 minutes

SERVES 4

GLUTEN-FREE NUT-FREE VEGAN

Brussels sprouts seem to be a polarizing vegetable that people either hate or love. I can almost guarantee that anyone who hates Brussels sprouts has never tried them roasted; the roasted nutty flavor the hot oven brings out is sure to be a new favorite. If you can buy the smallest Brussels sprouts in the batch, they are even better.

1 pound Brussels sprouts

2 tablespoons olive oil

1 tablespoon lemon juice

½ teaspoon salt

½ teaspoon freshly ground black pepper

1. Preheat the oven to 400°F. Line a baking sheet with foil.

2. On the prepared baking sheet, spread the Brussels sprouts in a single layer.

3. Drizzle the Brussels sprouts with the olive oil and lemon juice and sprinkle them with the salt and pepper.

4. Bake the Brussels sprouts for 30 minutes, checking to prevent burning, until they are tender with crispy edges.

Cooking tip: For crispier sprouts, peel back the leaves until you reach the centers, leaving more surface area to be baked to a crisp.

Per serving: Calories: 104; Total fat: 7g; Saturated fat: 1g; Cholesterol: 0mg; Sodium: 316mg; Carbohydrates: 9g; Fiber: 4g; Sugar: 2.5g; Protein: 3g

Succotash

Prep time: 5 minutes   Cook time: 20 minutes
SERVES 4
GLUTEN-FREE **NUT-FREE** ONE-POT **VEGAN**

Succotash is a corn-and-shell-bean dish popular in the summer for its refreshing flavors. It is often served with a whole grain and can include any variety of seasonal vegetables. This dish can be served warm or chilled and can even be used as a hearty salad topping.

1 (15-ounce) can no-salt-added lima beans, drained

1 (10-ounce) bag frozen corn

1 zucchini, quartered and diced

1 cup cherry tomatoes, halved

½ small red onion, diced

2 tablespoons white wine vinegar

2 tablespoons olive oil

1 tablespoon dried basil

1. In a large pot, cover the lima beans and frozen corn with water and cook on medium-high for 20 minutes. Drain the water.

2. Add the zucchini, tomatoes, onion, vinegar, olive oil, and basil and mix well.

3. Serve warm, or chill for 30 minutes and serve cold.

Substitution tip: Fresh or canned corn work equally well in this recipe! Frozen corn has wonderful flavor and has the added benefit of being available all year round. If you are craving a hint of summer during the colder months when fresh tomatoes are hard to find, use a can of diced tomatoes in place of the cherry tomatoes.

Per serving: Calories: 229; Total fat: 8.5g; Saturated fat: 1g; Cholesterol: 0mg; Sodium: 39mg; Carbohydrates: 34g; Fiber: 8g; Sugar: 4g; Protein: 9g

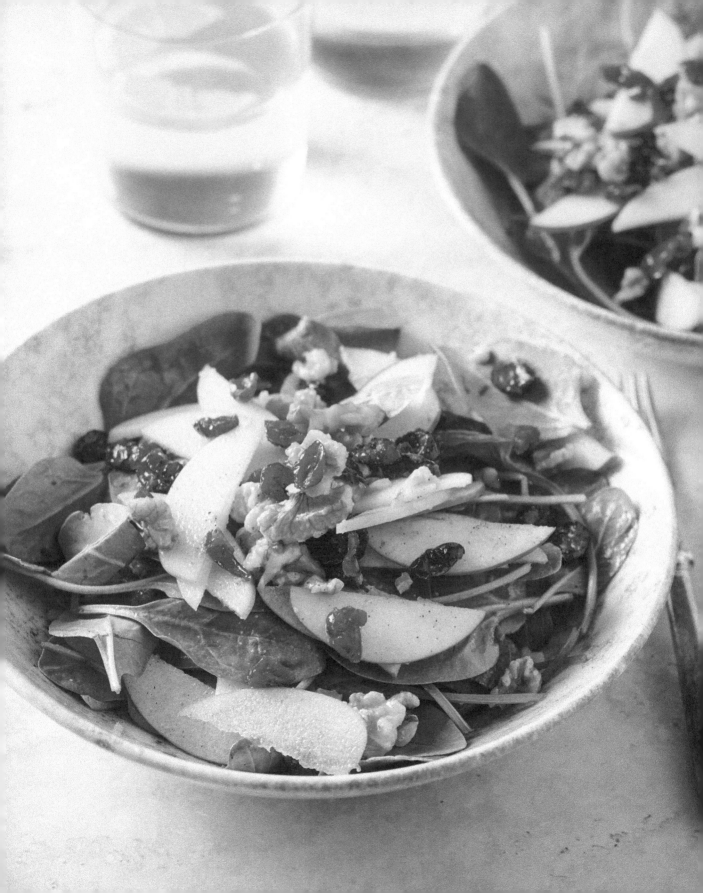

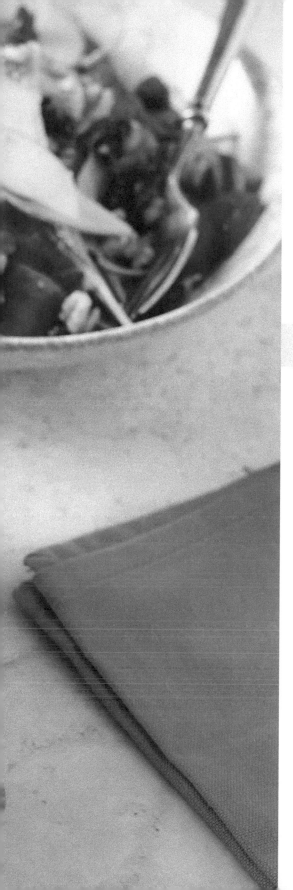

CHAPTER SIX

Salads and Vegetarian Mains

Apple, Walnut, and Spinach Salad

Prep time: 15 minutes
SERVES 4
CONTAINS NUTS GLUTEN-FREE VEGAN

I like to think of this salad as the apple pie of salads. It embodies the hallmarks of the all-American apple pie: delicious apples, warm flavors of cinnamon and nutmeg, and crunchy nuts.

8 cups baby spinach

2 medium apples, any variety, thinly sliced

1 cup walnut pieces

½ cup dried cranberries

¾ cup olive oil

¼ cup white wine vinegar

1 teaspoon ground cinnamon

½ teaspoon ground nutmeg

1. In a large bowl, combine the spinach, apples, walnuts, and cranberries until well mixed.

2. In a small bowl, whisk together the olive oil, vinegar, cinnamon, and nutmeg.

3. Serve each plate of salad with a drizzle of the dressing. Store the leftover dressing in an airtight container in the refrigerator for up to 2 weeks.

Variation tip: As prepared, this salad is vegan, but it would go wonderfully with shredded chicken or salmon.

Per serving (¼ salad + 2 tablespoons dressing): Calories: 508; Total fat: 41g; Saturated fat: 5g; Cholesterol: 0mg; Sodium: 89mg; Carbohydrates: 32g; Fiber: 8g; Sugar: 20g; Protein: 8g

Blueberry, Almond, and Kale Salad

Prep time: 15 minutes

SERVES 4

CONTAINS NUTS GLUTEN-FREE VEGAN

Kale is a hearty leafy-green vegetable that has more body than lettuce. It has a delightful chew that is satisfying and will keep you full for hours. This salad is jazzed up with bright blueberries and crunchy sliced almonds.

6 cups chopped kale

2 cups blueberries

1 cup sliced almonds

¼ red onion, thinly sliced

¾ cup olive oil

¼ cup lemon juice

1 teaspoon garlic powder

¼ teaspoon freshly
  ground black pepper

1. In a large bowl, combine the kale, blueberries, almonds, and onion until well mixed.

2. In a small bowl, whisk together the olive oil, lemon juice, garlic powder, and pepper.

3. Serve each salad with a drizzling of dressing. Store the leftover dressing in an airtight container in the refrigerator for up to 2 weeks.

Did you know? Kale is incredibly nutrient dense, containing high amounts of vitamins A, K, and C as well as manganese and essential trace nutrients like copper. It contains omega-3 fatty acids as well as high levels of antioxidants.

Per serving (¼ salad + 2 tablespoons dressing): Calories: 370; Total fat: 32g; Saturated fat: 3.5g; Cholesterol: 0mg; Sodium: 11mg; Carbohydrates: 19g; Fiber: 5.5g; Sugar: 9.5g; Protein: 7g

Avocado, Tomato, and Arugula Salad

Prep time: 15 minutes

SERVES 4

CONTAINS NUTS GLUTEN-FREE VEGAN

This salad has the best of all worlds—it's crisp, creamy, sweet, savory, bitter, and sour—and is loaded with healthy fat, which is essential for brain health. The avocado will help keep you full.

8 cups arugula

2 avocados, diced

2 cups diced tomatoes

⅔ cup olive oil

¼ cup lemon juice

2 tablespoons
  Dijon mustard

½ teaspoon garlic powder

¼ teaspoon freshly
  ground black pepper

1. In a large bowl, combine the arugula, avocados, and tomatoes until well mixed.

2. In a small bowl, whisk together the olive oil, lemon juice, mustard, garlic powder, and pepper.

3. Serve each salad with a drizzling of dressing. Store the leftover dressing in an airtight container in the refrigerator for up to 2 weeks.

Variation tip: The flavors in this salad would go perfectly with black beans, chicken, salmon, or shrimp.

Per serving (¼ salad + 2 tablespoons dressing): Calories: 331; Total fat: 30g; Saturated fat: 4g; Cholesterol: 0mg; Sodium: 216mg; Carbohydrates: 13g; Fiber: 7g; Sugar: 5g; Protein: 4g

Warm Romaine Salad

Prep time: 10 minutes   Cook time: 20 minutes

SERVES 4

NUT-FREE   VEGAN

A warm salad may sound different, but roasting vegetables in the oven gives them a rich, almost nutty flavor. This salad is tasty proof that you can enjoy leafy salad greens other ways than just cold!

2 cups cherry or grape tomatoes, halved

2 zucchini, cut into half-moons

2 cups cubed whole wheat bread

½ tablespoon jarred minced garlic

2 romaine lettuce hearts, halved lengthwise

¾ cup olive oil

¼ cup balsamic vinegar

1 tablespoon dried oregano

1. Preheat the oven to 400°F. Line a baking sheet or pan with foil.

2. On the prepared baking sheet, combine the tomatoes, zucchini, bread cubes, and garlic. Bake for 10 minutes, or until the zucchini are tender and the bread is beginning to brown.

3. Add the romaine hearts and bake everything together for 10 more minutes, until the lettuce begins to wilt.

4. While the vegetables are baking, in a small bowl, whisk together the olive oil, balsamic vinegar, and oregano.

5. Serve each romaine half with a scoop of tomatoes, zucchini, and bread and a drizzle of the dressing. Store the leftover dressing in an airtight container in the refrigerator for up to 2 weeks.

Cooking tip: This dish would also be easy to cook on a grill or on the stove in a grill pan. The char would add new depth to the flavor profile.

Per serving (¼ salad + 2 tablespoons dressing): Calories: 289; Total fat: 22g; Saturated fat: 3g; Cholesterol: 0mg; Sodium: 139mg; Carbohydrates: 20g; Fiber: 2g; Sugar: 6.5g; Protein: 4g

Berry Spring Greens

Prep time: 15 minutes
SERVES 4
CONTAINS NUTS   GLUTEN-FREE   VEGAN

This salad works beautifully with a piece of chicken or salmon, as the topping on a sandwich, or as a quick lunch. It is loaded with berries, making a crisp salad that will satisfy your sweet tooth, no dessert required.

8 cups spring greens

1 cup blueberries

1 cup raspberries

1 cup sliced strawberries

1 cup chopped nuts
of choice

¾ cup olive oil

¼ cup balsamic vinegar

¼ teaspoon garlic powder

¼ teaspoon freshly
ground black pepper

1. In a large bowl, combine the spring greens, blueberries, raspberries, strawberries, and nuts until well mixed.

2. In a small bowl, whisk together the olive oil, balsamic vinegar, garlic powder, and pepper.

3. Serve each salad with a drizzling of dressing. Store the leftover dressing in an airtight container in the refrigerator for up to 2 weeks.

Ingredient tip: You can use fresh fruit, thawed frozen fruit, or drained canned fruit in this recipe.

Per serving (¼ salad + 2 tablespoons dressing):
Calories: 443; Total fat: 40g; Saturated fat: 4.5g; Cholesterol: 0mg; Sodium: 74mg; Carbohydrates: 23g; Fiber: 7.5g; Sugar: 9g; Protein: 7g

Mediterranean Chard Salad

Prep time: 15 minutes

SERVES 4

CONTAINS NUTS GLUTEN-FREE VEGAN

This salad is directly inspired by the Mediterranean ingredients that inform much of the MIND diet. Mediterranean flavors include fresh fruits and vegetables, beans, olive oil, nuts, and herbs, all of which you will find here.

8 cups Swiss chard or rainbow chard, torn into bite-size pieces

1 (15-ounce) can chickpeas, drained

1 cucumber, cut into half-moons

1 cup grape or cherry tomatoes, halved

1 cup pine nuts

½ small red onion, thinly sliced

½ cup dried cranberries

¾ cup olive oil

¼ cup lemon juice

1 tablespoon dried basil

¼ teaspoon red pepper flakes

1. In a large bowl, combine the chard, chickpeas, cucumber, tomatoes, pine nuts, onion, and cranberries until well mixed.

2. In a small bowl, whisk together the olive oil, lemon juice, basil, and red pepper flakes.

3. Serve each salad with a drizzling of dressing. Store the leftover dressing in an airtight container in the refrigerator for up to 2 weeks.

Did you know? Chickpeas, also known as garbanzo beans, are high in protein, fiber, vitamins, minerals, and antioxidants. They are a very versatile bean—you can even make coffee from chickpeas!

Per serving (¼ salad + 2 tablespoons dressing): Calories: 573; Total fat: 45g; Saturated fat: 4.5g; Cholesterol: 0mg; Sodium: 305mg; Carbohydrates: 40g; Fiber: 8.5g; Sugar: 17g; Protein: 12g

Tuscan Bean Soup

Prep time: 10 minutes   Cook time: 20 minutes
SERVES 6
GLUTEN-FREE   NUT-FREE   ONE-POT   VEGAN

This broth-based soup is full of hearty ingredients like kale and cabbage as well as tender ingredients like carrots and cannellini beans. With a variety of textures and flavors, this classic homestyle soup is sure to satisfy. Serve with a side salad or a slice of crusty bread for dipping.

6 cups low-sodium vegetable stock

2 (15-ounce) cans no-salt-added cannellini beans, drained

2 cups shredded kale

2 cups shredded cabbage

2 cups diced celery

2 cups diced carrots

2 tablespoons tomato paste

1 tablespoon lemon juice

1 tablespoon dried oregano

½ tablespoon garlic powder

In a stockpot or another large and deep pot, combine the vegetable stock, beans, kale, cabbage, celery, carrots, tomato paste, lemon juice, oregano, and garlic powder. Cover and cook on medium-high for 20 minutes, until the carrots are tender. The soup will come to a boil.

Cooking tip: This soup makes wonderful leftovers to freeze. The ingredients are simple and inexpensive enough that you can easily double the recipe and freeze the leftovers for a rainy day.

Per serving: Calories: 180; Total fat: 1g; Saturated fat: 0g; Cholesterol: 0mg; Sodium: 217mg; Carbohydrates: 33g; Fiber: 11g; Sugar: 8g; Protein: 10g

One-Pot Lentils and Rice

Prep time: 5 minutes   Cook time: 25 minutes
SERVES 4
GLUTEN-FREE NUT-FREE ONE-POT VEGAN

Lentils are rich in fiber, protein, vitamins, and minerals and have long been a staple in the diets of many cultures around the world. When paired with rice, they are a complete vegan protein that is hearty and satisfying. Here nutrient-dense wild rice is used, which provides a nutty flavor and chewy texture along with antioxidants and added fiber.

6 cups water
2 cups brown lentils
2 carrots,
  coarsely chopped
1 cup wild rice
1 teaspoon ground thyme
1 teaspoon garlic powder
2 cups fresh spinach
1 lemon

1. In a stockpot or another large and deep pot, combine the water, lentils, carrots, wild rice, thyme, and garlic powder.

2. Bring to a high simmer over medium-high heat. Reduce the heat and simmer until the lentils and rice are tender, about 15 to 20 minutes.

3. During the last few minutes before serving, stir in the spinach and allow to wilt.

4. Halve the lemon and squeeze its juice into the pot and serve.

Ingredient tip: Before cooking, make sure to rinse lentils in a strainer to remove any sediment, checking for any small rocks or debris.

Per serving: Calories: 502; Total fat: 1.5g; Saturated fat: 0g; Cholesterol: 0mg; Sodium: 51mg; Carbohydrates: 95g; Fiber: 14g; Sugar: 4.5g; Protein: 30g

Green Chile Stew

Prep time: 10 minutes   Cook time: 20 minutes

SERVES 4

GLUTEN-FREE **NUT-FREE** ONE-POT **VEGAN**

Green chile stew is on my mind every single day. Here in Colorado, every family I know has its own rendition of this dish. This version can be served as a hearty stew or as a smother sauce for burritos.

1 (27-ounce) can whole green chiles

2 cups low-sodium vegetable stock

1 (15-ounce) can no-salt-added petite diced tomatoes

1 large white onion, diced

2 jalapeño peppers, seeded and diced

2 tablespoons jarred minced garlic

1 tablespoon chili powder

1 tablespoon ground cumin

1 tablespoon dried oregano

1. In a stockpot or another large and deep pot, combine the chiles and their juices, vegetable stock, tomatoes and their juices, onion, jalapeño, garlic, chili powder, cumin, and oregano and simmer over medium-high heat for 20 minutes, or until the onions and peppers are softened.

2. Serve warm.

Variation tip: You can add cooked chicken to this recipe for a delectable chicken green chile stew.

Per serving: Calories: 102; Total fat: 0g; Saturated fat: 0g; Cholesterol: 0mg; Sodium: 891mg; Carbohydrates: 21g; Fiber: 7g; Sugar: 9g; Protein: 6g

Chickpea Sliders

Prep time: 5 minutes   Cook time: 10 minutes
SERVES 4
NUT-FREE ONE-POT VEGAN

I made these sliders often when I was easing my husband into a more plant-based diet. They work really well in a picnic or as your lunch on a hike or biking day. Because they are cooked in the microwave and only require one bowl to make, they are perfect for a quick weeknight meal.

2 (15-ounce) cans no-salt-added chickpeas

1 large avocado, mashed

1 tablespoon olive oil

1 tablespoon lemon juice

1 teaspoon garlic powder

Freshly ground black pepper

4 whole wheat slider buns

1. In a medium microwave-safe bowl, microwave the chickpeas and their liquid for 10 minutes.

2. Drain most of the liquid from the bowl and mash most of the chickpeas with a fork or potato masher. You want some of the chickpeas to remain whole for texture.

3. Add the avocado, olive oil, lemon juice, garlic powder, and pepper to taste and mix well.

4. Serve each slider bun with one-quarter of the chickpea mixture.

Substitution tip: Swap in your favorite gluten-free buns or bread to make this recipe gluten-free.

Per serving: Calories: 397; Total fat: 14g; Saturated fat: 1g; Cholesterol: 0mg; Sodium: 160mg; Carbohydrates: 58g; Fiber: 14g; Sugar: 6.5g; Protein: 16g

Three-Bean Chili

Prep time: 5 minutes   Cook time: 25 minutes

SERVES 4

GLUTEN-FREE **NUT-FREE** ONE-POT **VEGAN**

Chili may not be anything fancy, and that is exactly the point. Classic comfort food has its place on the MIND diet. This chili is also an easy recipe for adding extra vegetables like carrots, sweet potatoes, and bell peppers. Serve with crackers or corn chips.

2 (15-ounce) cans no-salt-added tomato sauce

1 (15-ounce) can no-salt-added pinto beans, drained

1 (15-ounce) can no-salt-added black beans, drained

1 (15-ounce) can no-salt-added kidney beans, drained

1 (14.5-ounce) can no-salt-added petite diced tomatoes, drained

1 small white onion, finely diced

2 celery stalks, finely diced

3 tablespoons chili powder

1 tablespoon garlic powder

1½ teaspoons ground red pepper (optional)

In a large and deep pot, combine the tomato sauce, pinto beans, black beans, kidney beans, tomatoes, onion, celery, chili powder, garlic powder, and red pepper (if using), and cook over medium heat for 25 minutes, or until the beans and onions are tender.

Cooking tip: This recipe is a perfect freezer meal for a busy day; double or triple the recipe for inexpensive leftovers. Chili is one of those things that tends to taste better the next day!

Per serving: Calories: 416; Total fat: 2.5g; Saturated fat: 0g; Cholesterol: 0mg; Sodium: 348mg; Carbohydrates: 75g; Fiber: 25g; Sugar: 17g; Protein: 23g

Smothered Bean Burritos

Prep time: 5 minutes   Cook time: 25 minutes

SERVES 4

NUT-FREE VEGAN

A bean burrito (or tostada) is the go-to meal for me on a busy day, a lazy night, or when I do not feel like cooking. The best part is that it is MIND diet–friendly. If you happen to have any leftover Green Chile Stew (page 74), it is another great smother sauce that can be used in place of the sauce here.

FOR THE SAUCE

2 tablespoons olive oil

2 tablespoons
   all-purpose flour

1½ cups low-sodium
   vegetable stock

¼ cup chili powder

4 teaspoons chipotle
   chili powder

2 teaspoons
   ground cumin

1 teaspoon garlic powder

FOR THE BURRITOS

2 (15-ounce) cans
   no-salt-added black
   beans, drained

1 cup diced tomatoes,
   fresh or canned

1 teaspoon chili powder

¼ teaspoon garlic powder

4 whole wheat tortillas

TO MAKE THE SAUCE

1. In a medium pot, heat the olive oil over medium-high heat until shimmering. Sprinkle in the flour and mix until the flour has dissolved. Add the vegetable stock, chili powder, chipotle chili powder, cumin, and garlic powder and cook together over medium-low heat for 15 minutes, until the flavors combine.

TO MAKE THE BURRITOS

2. While the sauce is simmering, in a medium pot, combine the beans, tomatoes, chili powder, and garlic powder. Heat over medium heat for 20 minutes, or until the beans are tender.

3. To build each burrito, add one-quarter of the bean mixture to each tortilla, roll up, and smother with ½ cup of sauce.

Substitution tip: You can use any beans of your choice in these burritos. Whatever you have in the pantry will be perfect.

Per serving: Calories: 494; Total fat: 13g; Saturated fat: 3g; Cholesterol: 0mg; Sodium: 893mg; Carbohydrates: 75g; Fiber: 15g; Sugar: 4.5g; Protein: 18g

Zucchini Boats

Prep time: 10 minutes   Cook time: 20 minutes

SERVES 4

CONTAINS NUTS ONE-POT VEGAN

I like to think of these zucchini boats as an upgraded stuffed bell pepper. The zucchini provides a juicy and tender container for a hearty filling of black beans, greens, and tomatoes. Don't skip the pine nuts, which are a MIND diet superstar and bring a gentle nuttiness to the dish.

4 small to medium
   zucchini
2 tablespoons olive oil
1 (15-ounce) can
   no-salt-added black
   beans, drained
1 cup fresh or frozen
   chopped spinach
1 cup halved grape or
   cherry tomatoes
¼ cup pine nuts
1 tablespoon lemon juice
½ teaspoon red
   pepper flakes
½ cup panko
   bread crumbs

1. Preheat the oven to 350°F. Line a baking sheet with foil.

2. While the oven is preheating, cut each zucchini in half lengthwise and scoop out the seeds with a spoon, making a pocket down each zucchini half. On the prepared baking sheet, place each zucchini boat skin-side down.

3. Brush each zucchini boat with olive oil.

4. In a medium bowl, combine the beans, spinach, tomatoes, pine nuts, lemon juice, and red pepper flakes until well mixed.

5. Fill each of the zucchini halves with 4 to 6 tablespoons of the filling and sprinkle with the bread crumbs.

6. Roast the zucchini boats in the oven for 20 minutes, until the beans are tender.

Cooking tip: To speed up the process, this entire recipe can be prepared in the microwave, but you will miss a bit of the roasted flavor and crispiness.

Per serving: Calories: 287; Total fat: 14g; Saturated fat: 1.5g; Cholesterol: 0mg; Sodium: 72mg; Carbohydrates: 34g; Fiber: 8g; Sugar: 4.5g; Protein: 11g

Vegan Pesto Pasta

Prep time: 5 minutes   Cook time: 15 minutes

SERVES 4

CONTAINS NUTS VEGAN

Pesto is a traditional Italian sauce made by crushing pine nuts, garlic, basil leaves, hard cheese, and olive oil together with a mortar and pestle. It is easy to make variations of pesto with whatever you have on hand; just combine a leafy green, a nut, garlic, and olive oil. To make pesto vegan, simply omit cheese.

8 ounces whole wheat pasta, any shape

2 cups chopped fresh basil or 1 cup dried basil

½ cup olive oil

2 tablespoons pine nuts

2 teaspoons jarred minced garlic

1. Bring a large pot of water to a boil. Cook the pasta for 10 to 12 minutes, until tender. Drain.

2. While the pasta is cooking, in a bowl, combine the basil, olive oil, pine nuts, and garlic. Choose one of the following methods to continue:

   a)   On a large cutting board, use a rolling pin to repeatedly roll over the mixture, crushing it into a thick paste.

   b)   Pulse together in a blender to create a thick paste.

3. Add the pesto to the pasta and mix until all the pasta is well coated in the sauce.

> **Did you know?** The nutritional value of fresh and dried basil is virtually the same. If you cannot get your hands on fresh basil, you can always substitute dried basil. If you prefer having fresh, consider growing basil in a small pot at home.

Per serving: Calories: 505; Total fat: 33g; Saturated fat: 4.5g; Cholesterol: 0mg; Sodium: 8mg; Carbohydrates: 48g; Fiber: 6.5g; Sugar: 1.5g; Protein: 11g

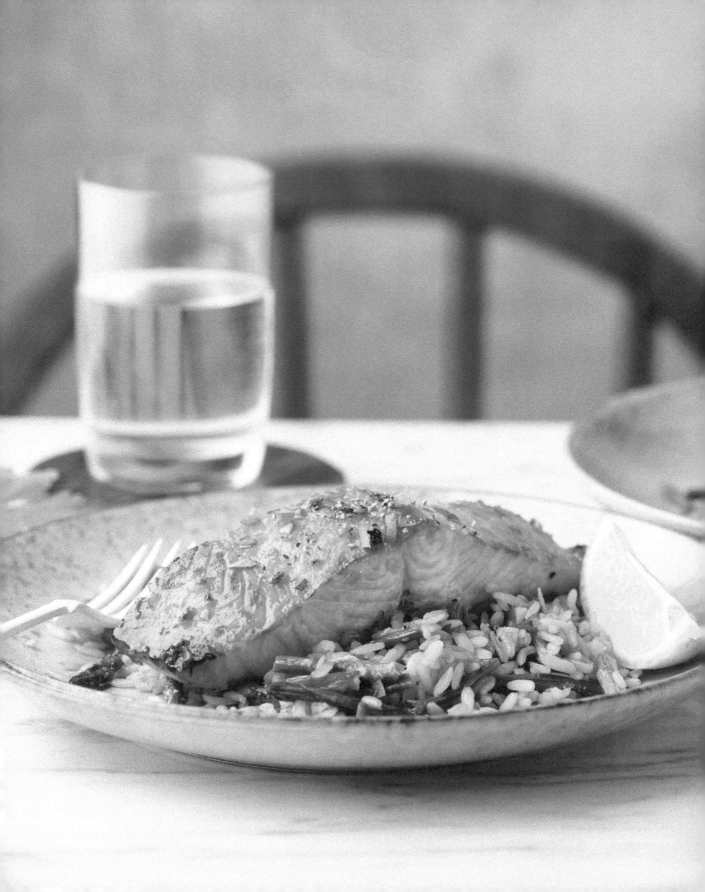

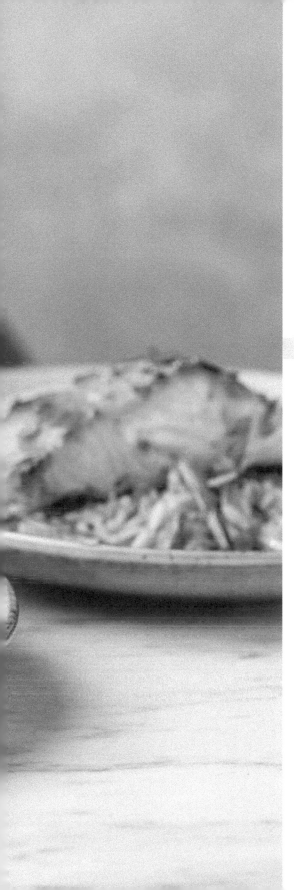

CHAPTER SEVEN

Seafood Mains

Fresh Tomato Shrimp Pasta

Prep time: 5 minutes   Cook time: 15 minutes

SERVES 4

NUT-FREE

This pasta dish is the trifecta—simple, quick, and delicious. What could be better? Fresh ingredients make the best meals, and this dish proves it. Make the shrimp, spinach, and tomato sauce while the noodles are cooking, and this dish will be nearly ready to eat by the time they are done.

8 ounces whole wheat spaghetti or linguine

2 tablespoons olive oil

8 ounces shrimp, raw or precooked, shells and tails removed

2 cups diced tomatoes

1 cup baby spinach

½ teaspoon jarred minced garlic

1. Bring a large pot of water to a boil. Cook the pasta for 10 to 12 minutes, until tender. Drain.

2. While the pasta is cooking, in a large pan, heat the olive oil over medium heat until shimmering. Add the shrimp, tomatoes, spinach, and garlic and cook together for 10 minutes, until the shrimp are pink and opaque.

3. Add the pasta to the pan of sauce and shrimp and toss together until well combined.

Ingredient tip: If you are not comfortable cooking raw shrimp, you can purchase precooked shrimp at the grocery store meat counter. Cooking them in this method will not overcook the shrimp or make them rubbery.

Per serving: Calories: 352; Total fat: 10g; Saturated fat: 1.5g; Cholesterol: 79mg; Sodium: 80mg; Carbohydrates: 51g; Fiber: 7.5g; Sugar: 3.5g; Protein: 20g

Roasted Pesto Trout

Prep time: 10 minutes   Cook time: 20 minutes
SERVES 4
CONTAINS NUTS GLUTEN-FREE

Trout are freshwater fish high in omega-3 fatty acids, B vitamins, potassium, and phosphorus. They have light pink flesh and are similar in flavor to salmon. Serve with salad, pasta, rice, or crusty bread.

2 cups chopped fresh basil or 1 cup dried basil

½ cup olive oil

2 tablespoons pine nuts

2 teaspoons jarred minced garlic

2 whole trout or 4 trout fillets

1. Preheat the oven to 400°F. Line a baking sheet with foil and set aside.

2. In a bowl, combine the basil, olive oil, pine nuts, and garlic. Choose one of the following methods to make your pesto:

   a) On a large cutting board, use a rolling pin to repeatedly roll over the mixture, crushing it into a thick paste.

   b) Pulse together in a blender to create a thick paste.

3. If using whole trout, stuff each trout with half of the pesto. If using trout fillets, coat each fillet with one-quarter of the pesto. Place the trout on the prepared baking sheet.

4. Bake the trout for 15 to 20 minutes, until the fish is opaque and flakes easily with a fork.

Ingredient tip: Ask the butcher to gut the trout for you, if they aren't already gutted. They will still contain bones; eat carefully around them or peel from the fillet after cooking.

Per serving: Calories: 392; Total fat: 35g; Saturated fat: 5g; Cholesterol: 46mg; Sodium: 43mg; Carbohydrates: 1g; Fiber: 0.5g; Sugar: 0g; Protein: 18g

Honey-Garlic Salmon

Prep time: 5 minutes   Cook time: 15 minutes
SERVES 4
GLUTEN-FREE NUT-FREE

This sheet pan dinner calls for fresh salmon, but you can easily use frozen fillets or even canned salmon in its place. The simple honey-garlic glazed salmon tastes amazing over pasta or a salad. I like to use this recipe as a basic blueprint for crafting a variety of different meals.

1 bunch asparagus

1 tablespoon olive oil

Freshly ground black pepper

1 pound skinless salmon fillets

2 tablespoons honey

1 teaspoon jarred minced garlic

1 (3.5-ounce) boil-in-bag brown rice

1. Preheat the oven to 400°F. Line a baking sheet with foil.

2. Cut the asparagus into bite-size pieces, place on the baking sheet, drizzle with olive oil, and season with pepper.

3. In a small bowl, combine the honey and garlic. Coat all sides of the salmon in the honey-and-garlic mixture and add it to the baking sheet.

4. Bake the asparagus and salmon in a single layer for 15 minutes, checking often to prevent burning. The honey-and-garlic mixture should caramelize the exterior of the salmon.

5. While the asparagus and salmon are baking, fill a large pot halfway with water and bring to a boil.

6. Cook the rice for 10 minutes, or according to the instructions on the package.

7. Serve the salmon and asparagus over a bed of rice.

Did you know? Honey contains powerful polyphenols—antioxidants that are key for brain health—and has other anti-inflammatory properties.

Per serving: Calories: 384; Total fat: 17g; Saturated fat: 3.5g; Cholesterol: 82mg; Sodium: 60mg; Carbohydrates: 30g; Fiber: 2g; Sugar: 9.5g; Protein: 28g

Cajun-Style Whitefish

Prep time: 10 minutes   Cook time: 10 minutes

SERVES 4

GLUTEN-FREE NUT-FREE

Cajun cuisine comes from Louisiana and is a vibrant blend of French, Spanish, and West African flavors. Cajun cooking relies on fresh, local ingredients, aromatic vegetables, and spices like the ones found in this whitefish recipe. Serve over salad, rice, or pasta.

1 tablespoon cornstarch

1 teaspoon garlic powder

1 teaspoon onion powder

1 teaspoon paprika

1 teaspoon freshly ground
black pepper

1 teaspoon dried oregano

1 teaspoon dried
thyme or ½ teaspoon
ground thyme

2 tablespoons olive oil

1 pound whitefish fillets
(tilapia, cod, snapper,
catfish)

1. In a large bowl, whisk together the cornstarch, garlic powder, onion powder, paprika, pepper, oregano, and thyme. Dredge the fish fillets in the mixture until well coated.

2. In a large pan, heat the olive oil over medium heat until shimmering.

3. Cook each side of the fillets for 5 minutes. Blackening of the exterior is desirable.

Variation tip: This blackening seasoning blend works on any fish, shrimp, and even chicken.

Per serving: Calories: 184; Total fat: 9g; Saturated fat: 1.5g; Cholesterol: 57mg; Sodium: 61mg; Carbohydrates: 4g; Fiber: 0.5g; Sugar: 0g; Protein: 23g

Loaded Shrimp Pasta

Prep time: 5 minutes   Cook time: 15 minutes
SERVES 4
NUT-FREE

Asparagus, peas, and mushrooms are delicious in this everything-but-the-kitchen-sink dish, but you can prepare the recipe using any vegetables you have on hand. With its sumptuous blend of sweet, savory, bitter, and acidic, get ready for this pasta to become a new favorite meal.

8 ounces whole wheat pasta

4 tablespoons olive oil

1 teaspoon jarred minced garlic

1 pound shrimp, peeled and deveined

1 bunch asparagus, cut into 1-inch pieces

1 cup fresh or frozen spinach

1 cup canned or frozen green peas

1 cup sliced mushrooms

1 cup cherry or grape tomatoes, halved

1 lemon, halved

1. Bring a large pot of water to a boil. Cook the pasta for 10 to 12 minutes, until tender. Drain.

2. While the pasta is cooking, in a large pan, heat the olive oil and garlic over medium heat until shimmering. Add the shrimp, asparagus, spinach, peas, mushrooms, and tomatoes, and cook for 10 minutes, until the shrimp are pink and opaque.

3. Add the pasta to the pan of shrimp and vegetables and toss together until well combined.

4. Serve with a squeeze of lemon juice.

Substitution tip: If you have a shellfish allergy, swap out the shrimp for canned tuna, flaked salmon, tofu, or chicken.

Per serving: Calories: 507; Total fat: 17g; Saturated fat: 2.5g; Cholesterol: 183mg; Sodium: 185mg; Carbohydrates: 58g; Fiber: 10g; Sugar: 5.5g; Protein: 37g

Balsamic Salmon

Prep time: 5 minutes   Cook time: 15 minutes

SERVES 4

GLUTEN-FREE NUT-FREE

Balsamic vinegar retains many of the nutrients in the grapes it is made from, including polyphenols and antioxidants that prevent oxidative cell damage and improve cardiovascular health. Serve this tangy, brain-friendly salmon on a bed of cooked greens, a salad, rice, or pasta.

4 tablespoons balsamic vinegar

1 tablespoon Dijon mustard

2 teaspoons dried rosemary

1 teaspoon honey

1 pound salmon fillets

1. Preheat the oven to 400°F. Line a baking sheet with foil and set aside.

2. In a bowl, combine the balsamic vinegar, mustard, rosemary, and honey. Coat the salmon in the sauce.

3. On the prepared baking sheet, bake the salmon for 15 minutes, checking to prevent burning, until the fish flakes easily with a fork. The balsamic sauce should caramelize the exterior of the salmon.

Variation tip: Tilapia, halibut, sea bass, and cod also taste amazing with balsamic vinegar.

Per serving: Calories: 207; Total fat: 8g; Saturated fat: 1g; Cholesterol: 72mg; Sodium: 150mg; Carbohydrates: 4g; Fiber: 0g; Sugar: 4g; Protein: 26g

Sweet Pepper Tilapia

Prep time: 5 minutes   Cook time: 15 minutes

SERVES 4

GLUTEN-FREE   NUT-FREE

Tilapia is an affordable, easy-to-find fish with a mild flavor that blends into many different dishes. It does not contain as many omega-3 fatty acids as other fish like salmon, sardines, or mackerel, but it is a great lean protein choice to add to your meal rotation.

FOR THE FISH

2 tablespoons olive oil

2 cups sweet cherry peppers, sliced

1 pound tilapia fillets

1 teaspoon sweet paprika

FOR THE DRESSING

2 tablespoons olive oil

1 tablespoon white wine vinegar

¼ teaspoon freshly ground black pepper

¼ teaspoon sweet paprika

TO MAKE THE FISH

1. In a medium pan or skillet, heat the olive oil over medium heat until shimmering. Cook the sweet peppers for 5 minutes, until heated through.

2. While the peppers are cooking, dust the tilapia fillets with the paprika.

3. Move the peppers to the side of the pan and add the tilapia to the pan. Sear for 5 minutes, flip the fillets, and sear the other side for 5 minutes, or until the fish is white and opaque.

TO MAKE THE DRESSING

4. While the fish is cooking, in a small bowl, whisk together the olive oil, vinegar, pepper, and paprika until well combined.

5. Serve each fillet drizzled with dressing.

Substitution tip: If you cannot find sweet cherry peppers, red, orange, or yellow bell peppers work well in this dish.

Per serving: Calories: 246; Total fat: 15g; Saturated fat: 2.5g; Cholesterol: 57mg; Sodium: 456mg; Carbohydrates: 2g; Fiber: 1g; Sugar: 1g; Protein: 24g

Chili-Lime Cod

Prep time: 5 minutes   Cook time: 15 minutes

SERVES 4

GLUTEN-FREE   NUT-FREE

Cod is a tender whitefish that is rich in omega-3 fatty acids. It is often used in fish fries like fish and chips, but with its buttery texture, it does not need to be deep-fried to taste great. It pairs wonderfully with fresh and acidic ingredients like lime in this baked preparation. Serve with black beans and rice or atop a salad.

1 tablespoon olive oil

1 tablespoon lime juice

1 teaspoon chili powder

½ teaspoon ground cumin

½ teaspoon dried cilantro

¼ teaspoon ground
  cayenne pepper

1 pound cod fillets

1. Preheat the oven to 400°F. Line a baking sheet with foil and set aside.

2. In a bowl, combine the olive oil, lime juice, chili powder, cumin, cilantro, and cayenne pepper. Coat the cod fillets in the paste.

3. Place the fillets on the prepared baking sheet and bake for 15 minutes, until the fish is white and opaque, checking to prevent burning.

Did you know? The flavonoids in citrus fruits help maintain healthy brain tissue, reduce inflammation, and maintain proper blood flow in the brain.

Per serving: Calories: 113; Total fat: 4g; Saturated fat: 0.5g; Cholesterol: 43mg; Sodium: 61mg; Carbohydrates: 0g; Fiber: 0g; Sugar: 0g; Protein: 18g

Avocado Tuna Salad

Prep time: 5 minutes
SERVES 4
GLUTEN-FREE **NUT-FREE** ONE-POT

Tuna salad does not have to be the standard mayonnaise, mustard, and pickle relish mixture. The creaminess in this healthy variation is provided by avocado rather than mayonnaise and is paired with the brightness of bell pepper and the crispness of celery. Serve over salad, on your favorite bread, in a wrap, or on crackers.

2 (5-ounce) cans chunk
   light tuna, drained
1 large avocado, mashed
1 red bell pepper,
   finely diced
2 celery stalks,
   finely diced
1 tablespoon lemon or
   lime juice
Freshly ground
   black pepper

In a medium bowl, combine the tuna, avocado, bell pepper, celery, lemon juice, and pepper to taste until well mixed.

Did you know? Canned tuna is an excellent, affordable option to add omega-3 fatty acids to your diet. You may be concerned that canned tuna contains mercury, which many fish do. Choosing chunk light tuna over chunk white or solid albacore reduces mercury content. The rule of thumb is that women can safely consume 12.5 ounces of tuna per week and men 14.5 ounces per week. (A standard can of tuna is 5 ounces.)

Per serving: Calories: 154; Total fat: 8.5g; Saturated fat: 1.5g; Cholesterol: 24mg; Sodium: 260mg; Carbohydrates: 6g; Fiber: 3g; Sugar: 1.5g; Protein: 14g

Shrimp Tacos

Prep time: 10 minutes   Cook time: 15 minutes

SERVES 4

GLUTEN-FREE NUT-FREE

Shrimp tacos are a fresh, versatile alternative to ground beef tacos. Depending on your preference, you can use fresh, frozen, or canned shrimp for your filling. Shrimp is a lean protein option that is also rich in omega-3 and omega-6 fatty acids.

1 tablespoon olive oil

1 pound shrimp, peeled and deveined

1 teaspoon dried oregano

⅛ teaspoon chili powder

⅛ teaspoon garlic powder

⅛ teaspoon onion powder

1 cup plain coleslaw mix or shredded cabbage

1 small tomato, diced

1 tablespoon lime juice

8 corn tortillas

1. In a medium pan or skillet, heat the olive oil over medium heat until shimmering.

2. In a large bowl, toss the shrimp with the oregano, chili powder, garlic powder, and onion powder.

3. Cook the shrimp for 2 to 3 minutes per side, or until they are opaque and pink.

4. While the shrimp are cooking, in a medium bowl, combine the coleslaw mix, tomato, and lime juice. Set aside.

5. Remove the shrimp from the pan and allow them to rest while cooking the tortillas.

6. Wipe the pan with a paper towel and reuse it on high heat to heat the corn tortillas in small batches. Cook each tortilla for 1 minute per side, until they begin to brown.

7. Build each taco by filling the corn tortillas with shrimp and topping them with the coleslaw garnish.

Variation tip: Shrimp tacos can be topped with anything! For an alternative to coleslaw, top these tasty tacos with shredded lettuce, mixed spring greens, or baby spinach. Pico de gallo made with Roma tomato, finely diced onion, and jalapeño would also be a flavorful addition. Guacamole (page 52) would bring some nice creaminess to these simple, delicious tacos.

Per serving: Calories: 205; Total fat: 5g; Saturated fat: 0.5g; Cholesterol: 183mg; Sodium: 140mg; Carbohydrates: 16g; Fiber: 1.5g; Sugar: 1g; Protein: 25g

Dijon Salmon

Prep time: 5 minutes   Cook time: 15 minutes

SERVES 4

GLUTEN-FREE   NUT-FREE

Salmon—a fatty fish rich in anti-inflammatory omega-3s—pairs beautifully with both sweet and savory preparations. This recipe is a mix of both, featuring a honey Dijon mustard glaze that caramelizes while it bakes. Serve with rice, pasta, or vegetables.

1 tablespoon
 Dijon mustard

1 tablespoon honey

1 teaspoon lemon juice

¼ teaspoon
 ground thyme

12 ounces boneless,
 skinless salmon fillets

1. Preheat the oven to 450°F. Line a small baking dish with foil and set aside.

2. In a small bowl, whisk together the mustard, honey, lemon juice, and thyme.

3. Pat the salmon dry and place in the prepared baking dish.

4. Spread the honey mustard mixture on top of the salmon.

5. Bake uncovered for 12 to 15 minutes, or until the salmon reaches an internal temperature of 145°F and flakes easily with a fork.

Cooking tip: You can also panfry the salmon by cooking it for 4 minutes per side to give the fish a tasty crispy exterior.

Per serving: Calories: 158; Total fat: 6g; Saturated fat: 1g; Cholesterol: 54mg; Sodium: 133mg; Carbohydrates: 4g; Fiber: 0g; Sugar: 4.5g; Protein: 19g

Not Your Mother's Tuna Casserole

Prep time: 5 minutes   Cook time: 25 minutes
SERVES 4
NUT-FREE

Canned tuna is a MIND diet powerhouse. This tuna casserole is a warm, cozy option for integrating tuna into your repertoire when you aren't craving a tuna salad sandwich. This version amps up the flavor with earthy veggies like zucchini, mushrooms, and peas, bringing a healthy twist to a homestyle classic.

8 ounces whole wheat pasta (like penne or rotini)

2 (5-ounce) cans chunk light tuna, drained

1 cup shredded zucchini or squash

1 cup canned, fresh, or frozen peas

1 cup sliced mushrooms

1 (8-ounce) can no-salt-added tomato sauce

1 tablespoon fresh basil or ½ tablespoon dried basil

½ cup panko bread crumbs

Olive oil

1. Preheat the oven to 400°F.

2. Bring a large pot of water to a boil. Cook the pasta for 10 to 12 minutes, until tender. Drain.

3. While the pasta is cooking, in a 9-by-12-inch baking dish, combine the tuna, zucchini, peas, mushrooms, tomato sauce, and basil. Add the drained pasta to the pan and mix the ingredients together.

4. Top the casserole with the panko bread crumbs and a drizzle of olive oil.

5. Bake for 15 minutes to heat thoroughly and brown the panko bread crumbs.

Cooking tip: This is the perfect dish to utilize excess cooked pasta and veggies from the week.

Per serving: Calories: 470; Total fat: 13g; Saturated fat: 2g; Cholesterol: 24mg; Sodium: 325mg; Carbohydrates: 66g; Fiber: 9g; Sugar: 6.5g; Protein: 27g

Herbed Salmon Patties

Prep time: 10 minutes   Cook time: 10 minutes

SERVES 4

NUT-FREE

My dad always made the best fish patties, and I have created this recipe to celebrate my childhood. My dad's fish patties were always perfectly crispy and browned on the outside and flaky and soft on the inside. This dish replicates those same wonderful textures. I love these on their own, but they also make excellent burgers. Serve on a bun with your favorite condiments.

2 (5-ounce) cans salmon, drained

½ cup diced celery

⅓ cup panko bread crumbs, bread crumbs, or crushed unsalted saltine crackers

2 teaspoons chopped fresh dill or 1 teaspoon dried dill

1 teaspoon dried rosemary

1 teaspoon dried thyme

1 teaspoon lemon juice

Nonstick cooking spray

1. In a medium bowl, mash the salmon with a fork to achieve a flaked texture. Add the celery, panko bread crumbs, dill, rosemary, thyme, and lemon juice. With gloved or clean hands, blend the mixture together until all ingredients are well incorporated.

2. On a cutting board or flat food-safe surface, form 4 patties, each using one-quarter of the mixture.

3. Warm a large pan or skillet over medium heat. Spray the pan with cooking spray and sear each side of the patties for 3 to 5 minutes, to your preferred level of crispiness.

Substitution tip: You can use this exact preparation but substitute canned tuna or canned sardines. (Even if you are not a sardine fan, I urge you to give them a try.)

Per serving: Calories: 107; Total fat: 3g; Saturated fat: 0.5g; Cholesterol: 36mg; Sodium: 248mg; Carbohydrates: 6g; Fiber: 0.5g; Sugar: 0g; Protein: 15g

Lemon Sardine Pasta

Prep time: 5 minutes   Cook time: 15 minutes
SERVES 4
NUT-FREE

Canned sardines, which do not require any additional cooking, make a salty, protein-rich snack or a simple addition to a pasta or salad. They are high in omega-3 fatty acids, calcium, iron, and B vitamins and can be purchased skinless and boneless, though both the skin and bones are edible.

8 ounces whole wheat spaghetti

4 cups baby spinach

2 (3.75-ounce) cans sardines, drained

2 tablespoons olive oil

2 tablespoons jarred minced garlic

1 tablespoon lemon juice

1. Bring a large pot of water to a boil. Cook the pasta for 10 to 12 minutes, until tender. Drain.

2. During the last 5 minutes of cooking the pasta, add the spinach to the pot to cook. Drain the water.

3. While the pasta is cooking, in a large and deep pan or skillet, over medium heat, combine the sardines, olive oil, garlic, and lemon juice. Cook together for 5 minutes, until the flavors have combined to create a sauce.

4. Add the pasta and spinach to the sardine pan sauce and toss together until evenly coated.

Ingredient tip: Sardines are commonly purchased in the can and come packed in water, oil, or tomato sauce. All these options work well in this recipe; taste-test a few varieties to discover your favorite.

Per serving: Calories: 414; Total fat: 15g; Saturated fat: 2g; Cholesterol: 70mg; Sodium: 203mg; Carbohydrates: 50g; Fiber: 7.5g; Sugar: 1.5g; Protein: 23g

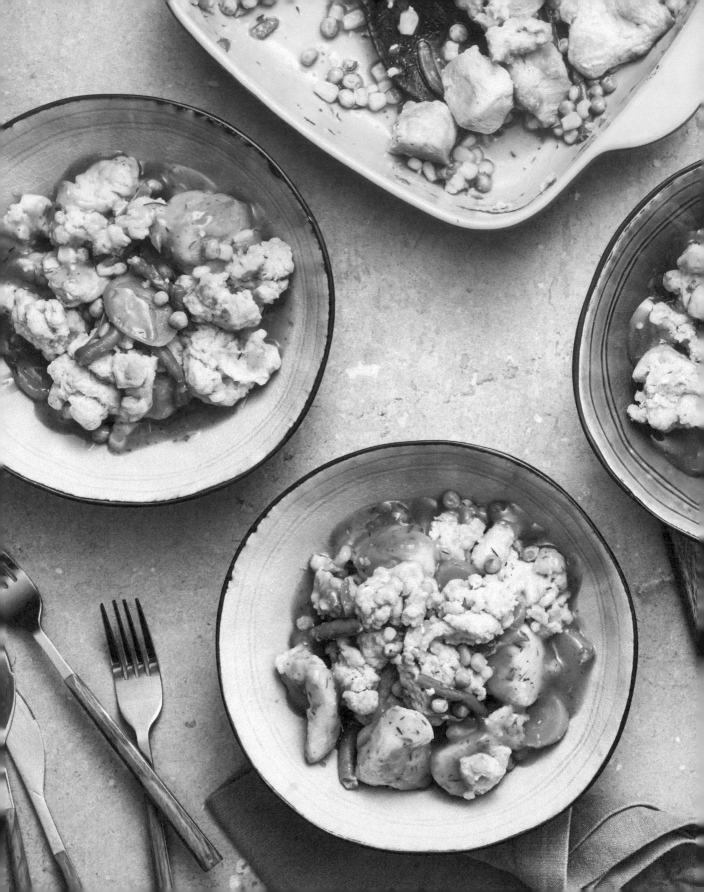

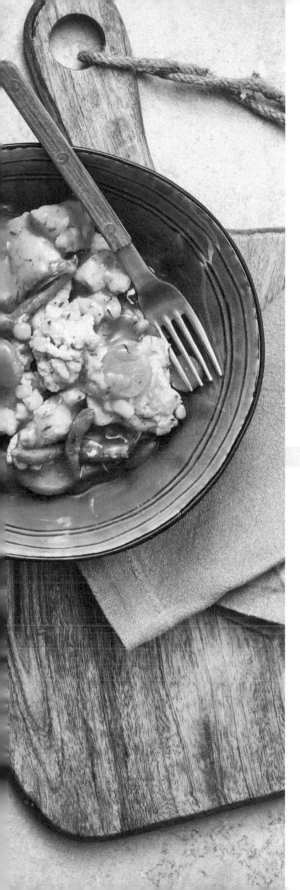

CHAPTER EIGHT

Poultry Mains

Chicken Enchiladas

Prep time: 10 minutes   Cook time: 20 minutes
SERVES 4
GLUTEN-FREE NUT-FREE

Enchilada literally means "decorated with chiles," a fitting name for this spicy, rich dish. Enchiladas invite all kinds of variation; try this recipe as is, and then experiment with any combination of vegetables, beans, and meats. Smother in a chili powder–flavored sauce, and you have a delicious plate of enchiladas! Serve with a salad, and top with salsa or Guacamole (page 52).

1 (14.5-ounce) can no-salt-added diced fire-roasted tomatoes

1 tablespoon chili powder

1 tablespoon dried oregano

1 teaspoon chipotle chili powder

1 teaspoon garlic powder

1 teaspoon onion powder

8 corn tortillas

8 ounces precooked or canned chicken breast

1 (15-ounce) can no-salt-added pinto or black beans, drained

1 zucchini, diced

1. Preheat the oven to 350°F.

2. In a medium bowl, combine the tomatoes and their juices, chili powder, oregano, chipotle powder, garlic powder, and onion powder to create your sauce.

3. On a cutting board or clean surface, lay out the tortillas and fill each with a scoop of chicken, beans, and zucchini.

4. Roll each tortilla into a burrito shape. In a baking dish, line up the rolled enchiladas.

5. Cover the enchiladas in the sauce, and bake for 20 minutes.

Variation tip: With this recipe, your options are endless, and swaps can be made to match any preference. For example, my husband prefers flour tortillas, while I prefer green sauce. For more variety, replace the chicken with turkey, shrimp, tilapia, or a mixture of vegetables and beans.

Per serving (without toppings): Calories: 289; Total fat: 4.5g; Saturated fat: 0.5g; Cholesterol: 57mg; Sodium: 390mg; Carbohydrates: 36g; Fiber: 7.5g; Sugar: 4.5g; Protein: 26g

Thai-Inspired Peanut Chicken Pasta

Prep time: 5 minutes   Cook time: 15 minutes

SERVES 4

CONTAINS NUTS GLUTEN-FREE

Peanuts are not just for baseball games and PB and J sandwiches. They add a decadent, rich flavor to savory dishes and are particularly at home in Thai cooking. Peanuts are also a wonderful source of antioxidants, protein, fiber, vitamins, and minerals.

2 tablespoons olive oil

1 pound boneless, skinless chicken breast, cubed

4 tablespoons creamy peanut butter

4 tablespoons white or rice vinegar

2 tablespoons reduced-sodium soy sauce

6 ounces rice noodles

2 tablespoons chopped scallions, green part only, or chives

2 tablespoons crushed peanuts

Lime juice (optional)

1. In a large pan or skillet, heat the olive oil over medium heat until shimmering. Add the cubed chicken and cook for 5 to 7 minutes, until cooked through.

2. While the chicken is cooking, in a small bowl, whisk together the peanut butter, vinegar, and soy sauce and set aside.

3. Bring a medium pot of water to a boil. Cook the rice noodles for 2 to 3 minutes, until tender. Drain.

4. Add the noodles to the pan of chicken. Add the peanut butter sauce and stir well to combine all ingredients.

5. Top with the scallions, peanuts, and lime juice (if using) and serve.

Substitution tip: You can replace the peanut butter with almond butter, sunflower seed butter, or tahini depending on your sensitivities and flavor preferences.

Per serving: Calories: 473; Total fat: 21g; Saturated fat: 3.5g; Cholesterol: 83mg; Sodium: 424mg; Carbohydrates: 39g; Fiber: 2g; Sugar: 2g; Protein: 33g

Jambalaya

Prep time: 5 minutes   Cook time: 30 minutes

SERVES 4

GLUTEN-FREE NUT-FREE

Jambalaya is a Louisiana-Cajun dish, similar to paella, with a tomato base and often including a variety of meats. Here, chicken provides a lean source of protein and a nice base for the flavorful sauce.

2 cups water

1 cup brown rice

2 tablespoons olive oil

8 ounces boneless, skinless chicken breast, cubed

2 celery stalks, diced

1 green bell pepper, diced

1 small white or yellow onion, diced

2 bay leaves

1 (8-ounce) can no-salt-added tomato sauce

¼ teaspoon ground thyme

1. In a medium pot, bring the water and rice to a boil over high heat. Reduce the heat to low, cover the pot, and cook for 15 to 20 minutes, or until the rice can be fluffed with a fork.

2. While the rice is cooking, in a large pan, heat the olive oil over medium heat until shimmering. Add the chicken and cook for 5 to 7 minutes, until cooked through.

3. Add the celery, bell pepper, onion, and bay leaves to the pan and cook for 5 to 10 minutes, until the veggies are tender.

4. Add the cooked rice to the pan and stir to combine.

5. Add the tomato sauce and thyme to the pan and simmer for 10 minutes, until the flavors meld.

6. Remove the bay leaves and serve.

> **Did you know?** In Cajun cooking, celery, green bell pepper, and onion are called the "holy trinity," inspired by the Catholic roots of the culture. With high levels of antioxidants, this combination is also a MIND diet holy trinity.

Per serving: Calories: 357; Total fat: 10g; Saturated fat: 1.5g; Cholesterol: 41mg; Sodium: 68mg; Carbohydrates: 48g; Fiber: 4.5g; Sugar: 5g; Protein: 19g

Turkey Meat Loaf

Prep time: 10 minutes   Cook time: 20 minutes
SERVES 4
NUT-FREE

Enjoy this recipe as a fresh take on the comforting homestyle classic meat loaf. This healthy spin on the hearty entrée uses turkey instead of beef to reduce the saturated fat content and also includes savory vegetables like mushrooms to boost antioxidants and moisture. Serve the meat loaf with salad or a baked potato or as a sandwich on whole-grain toast.

1 tablespoon olive oil

1 pound lean
   ground turkey

2 cups button
   mushrooms, minced

**1 cup panko
   bread crumbs**

1 small white
   onion, minced

1 bunch fresh
   parsley, minced

⅓ cup low-sodium
   chicken stock

2 tablespoons ketchup

1 tablespoon
   Worcestershire sauce

1. Preheat the oven to 350°F. Line a loaf pan with parchment paper and set aside.

2. In a large pan or skillet, heat the olive oil over medium heat until shimmering. Parcook the ground turkey in the pan for 10 minutes, browning it slightly.

3. In a large bowl, combine the parcooked turkey, mushrooms, panko bread crumbs, onion, parsley, chicken stock, ketchup, and Worcestershire sauce. Using clean or gloved hands, mash the mixture together until all the ingredients are evenly distributed.

4. Pack the mixture into the loaf pan in a loaf shape.

5. Bake the meat loaf for 10 minutes, until it reaches an internal temperature of 165°F

6. Slice the meat loaf into 2-inch slices and serve.

Substitution tip: Ground chicken will work well in place of the ground turkey in this recipe.

Per serving: Calories: 304; Total fat: 12g; Saturated fat: 3g; Cholesterol: 81mg; Sodium: 286mg; Carbohydrates: 24g; Fiber: 1.5g; Sugar: 4.5g; Protein: 26g

Turkey Faux Roast

Prep time: 5 minutes   Cook time: 25 minutes

SERVES 8

GLUTEN-FREE **NUT-FREE** ONE-POT

This recipe takes only 30 minutes to create a delicious roast that would otherwise take all day. Though it tastes like it took forever, this roast is very practical for busy weeknights. Package the leftovers once they have cooled for several freezer meals.

2 pounds turkey breast, skinless if possible

2 sweet potatoes, peeled and diced

2 celery stalks, chopped

1 yellow onion, diced

2 tablespoons Dijon mustard

2 teaspoons ground thyme

1. In a large and deep pot or pan, combine the turkey, sweet potatoes, celery, onion, mustard, and thyme.

2. Add enough water to just cover the turkey and vegetables.

3. Cover and cook on high for 25 minutes. The boiling liquid will quickly stew the turkey and vegetables until the flavors blend.

4. Serve the turkey and vegetables with a generous spoonful of the cooking liquid.

Variation tip: In place of sweet potatoes and celery, you can use leftover vegetables from the week, reducing food waste and increasing your veggie intake.

Per serving: Calories: 159; Total fat: 0.5g; Saturated fat: 0g; Cholesterol: 45mg; Sodium: 216mg; Carbohydrates: 8g; Fiber: 1.5g; Sugar: 2g; Protein: 29g

Chicken Biscuit Casserole

Prep time: 10 minutes   Cook time: 25 minutes

SERVES 4

NUT-FREE

Biscuits are an ultimate comfort food for me. I'm crazy about their flaky texture, tender chew, and homey flavor. This recipe, which is loaded with healthy veggies and juicy chicken, is a prime example of preparing a comfort food in a MIND diet–friendly way.

2 cups all-purpose flour

¾ cup unsweetened plain
   nondairy milk

½ cup canola oil

1½ teaspoons
   baking powder

Nonstick cooking spray

1 pound boneless, skinless
   chicken breast, cubed

1 cup low-sodium
   chicken stock

1 tablespoon cornstarch

1 teaspoon garlic powder

1 teaspoon dried thyme

12 ounces frozen
   mixed vegetables or
   1 (15-ounce) can mixed
   vegetables, drained

1. Preheat the oven to 400°F.

2. In a large bowl, combine the flour, nondairy milk, canola oil, and baking powder. It is easiest to mix with clean or gloved hands. Set aside.

3. In a large pan or skillet over medium heat sprayed with cooking oil, cook the chicken for 5 to 7 minutes, or until cooked through.

4. In a measuring cup or small bowl, whisk together the chicken stock, cornstarch, garlic powder, and thyme.

5. In an 8-by-8 baking dish, combine the cooked chicken, mixed vegetables, and sauce. Cover the casserole with spoonfuls of the biscuit mixture, like making drop biscuits.

6. Bake for 15 minutes until the biscuits begin to brown and the casserole is bubbling.

> **Cooking tip:** Use canned chicken to shorten prep time even further.

Per serving: Calories: 698; Total fat: 32g; Saturated fat: 3g; Cholesterol: 83mg; Sodium: 125mg; Carbohydrates: 63g; Fiber: 4g; Sugar: 4.5g; Protein: 35g

Chicken Potpie

Store-bought frozen potpies take at least 15 minutes to reheat. Here, you can make this comfort food classic from scratch, with healthier ingredients, in only 30 minutes.

1¼ cups all-purpose flour

⅓ cup olive oil, plus
   1 tablespoon

3 tablespoons cold water

1 pound boneless, skinless
   chicken breast, cubed

1 cup low-sodium
   chicken stock

1 tablespoon cornstarch

1 teaspoon garlic powder

½ teaspoon freshly
   ground black pepper

1 (12-ounce) bag frozen
   green beans

1 cup sliced mushrooms

1. Preheat the oven to 400°F.

2. In a large bowl, combine the flour, ⅓ cup of olive oil, and water and mix with clean or gloved hands to form a ball. If the dough is too crumbly, you can add 1 more tablespoon of cold water. Roll the dough out into an 8-by-8-inch flat shape.

3. In a large pan or skillet, heat the remaining 1 tablespoon of olive oil over medium heat until shimmering. Add the cubed chicken and cook for 5 to 7 minutes, until cooked through.

4. In a measuring cup or small bowl, whisk together the chicken stock, cornstarch, garlic powder, and pepper.

5. In an 8-by-8-inch baking dish, combine the cooked chicken, green beans, mushrooms, and sauce. Cover the mixture with the pie dough, pinching over the edges to seal the pie dough.

6. Bake for 15 minutes, until the dough begins to brown and the casserole is bubbling.

Variation tip: Ground turkey works equally well. Canned chicken or precooked shredded chicken are options if you need to speed this recipe up.

Per serving: Calories: 672; Total fat: 42g; Saturated fat: 6g; Cholesterol: 83mg; Sodium: 76mg; Carbohydrates: 39g; Fiber: 3.5g; Sugar: 3g; Protein: 32g

Barbecue Platter

Prep time: 10 minutes   Cook time: 20 minutes
SERVES 4
GLUTEN-FREE **NUT-FREE** ONE-POT

You do not need a fancy grill or smoker to enjoy delectable barbecue flavors. Using a sheet pan, the oven, and fresh ingredients, you will have a crowd-pleasing platter of meat and vegetables in 30 minutes. Making your own five-ingredient barbecue sauce is quick and easy and allows you to create a healthier version without all the added sugars in just minutes.

1 pound boneless, skinless chicken breast, cubed

1 bunch asparagus, cut into 1-inch pieces

2 zucchini, cut into dials or strips

1 red bell pepper, sliced

1 red onion, sliced

1 (8-ounce) can no-salt-added tomato sauce

2 tablespoons vinegar

2 tablespoons honey

½ teaspoon garlic powder

½ teaspoon onion powder

1. Preheat the oven to 400°F. Line a baking sheet with foil.

2. Combine the chicken, asparagus, zucchini, bell pepper, and onion on the prepared baking sheet.

3. In a small bowl, whisk together the tomato sauce, vinegar, honey, garlic powder, and onion powder.

4. Drizzle the chicken and vegetables with the barbecue sauce and bake for 20 minutes until the vegetables are tender and the chicken is cooked through.

Did you know? Store-bought barbecue sauce contains high amounts of corn syrup, salt, and additives. This homemade barbecue sauce has a better flavor and is MIND diet-friendly.

Per serving. Calories: 225; Total fat: 3g; Saturated fat: 1g; Cholesterol: 63mg; Sodium: 85mg; Carbohydrates: 23g; Fiber: 4g; Sugar: 17g; Protein: 27g

Lasagna Bake

Prep time: 5 minutes   Cook time: 25 minutes

SERVES 4

NUT-FREE   ONE-PAN

The key to this recipe is to use oven-ready lasagna noodles. You can find them at any grocer right next to the regular lasagna noodles. Using oven-ready pasta means you do not have to boil the noodles first, drastically speeding up the cooking process.

1 tablespoon olive oil

8 ounces boneless, skinless chicken breast, diced

1 (28-ounce) can no-salt-added tomato sauce

1 zucchini, peeled, seeded, and diced

1 cup button mushrooms, diced

1 tablespoon dried oregano or Italian seasoning

1 teaspoon garlic powder

12 ounces oven-ready lasagna noodles (about 15 noodles)

1. Preheat the oven to 375°F.

2. In a medium pan or skillet, heat the olive oil over medium heat until shimmering.

3. Brown the chicken breast for 3 to 5 minutes, until the outside surface is opaque.

4. In a large bowl, combine the chicken, tomato sauce, zucchini, mushrooms, oregano, and garlic powder and mix well.

5. In a 9-by-12-inch baking dish, add one-third of the chicken and vegetable filling, pushing it to all the edges of the pan, and cover with 5 noodles. Repeat by adding one-third of the mixture covered with 5 noodles. Repeat one last time with the remaining mixture and the 5 remaining noodles.

6. Cover with aluminum foil and bake for 25 minutes.

Variation tip: This recipe can be made vegetarian by omitting the chicken and loading up with sliced vegetables instead.

Per serving: Calories: 499; Total fat: 6.5g; Saturated fat: 1g; Cholesterol: 31mg; Sodium: 96mg; Carbohydrates: 81g; Fiber: 7g; Sugar: 14g; Protein: 26g

Turkey Stroganoff

Prep time: 5 minutes   Cook time: 25 minutes
SERVES 4
NUT-FREE

Traditional beef stroganoff is a Russian-inspired dish featuring beef in a rich sour cream sauce. To make this dish MIND diet–friendly, we are using ground turkey and going dairy-free while still maintaining the creamy texture and savory flavor profile that makes beef stroganoff a favorite.

8 ounces whole wheat pasta, like penne or rigatoni

1 tablespoon olive oil

1 pound lean ground turkey

2 cups unsweetened plain nondairy milk

8 ounces button mushrooms, sliced

2 tablespoons Dijon mustard

1 tablespoon Worcestershire sauce

¼ cup low-sodium chicken stock

2 tablespoons cornstarch

2 tablespoons dried parsley

1. Bring a large pot of water to a boil. Cook the pasta for 10 to 12 minutes, until tender. Drain.

2. While the pasta is cooking, in a large pan or skillet, heat the olive oil over medium heat until shimmering. Add the ground turkey and cook for 10 minutes, until the meat begins to brown.

3. Raise the heat to medium-high and add the nondairy milk, mushrooms, mustard, and Worcestershire sauce to the ground turkey. Cook for 10 minutes.

4. In a small bowl, whisk together the chicken stock, cornstarch, and parsley.

5. While stirring the turkey mixture, stir in the cornstarch slurry and cook together for 5 minutes.

6. Allow the dish to cool and thicken for a few minutes before serving.

Substitution tip: To make this recipe gluten-free, serve over brown rice instead of pasta.

Per serving: Calories: 486; Total fat: 15g; Saturated fat: 3.5g; Cholesterol: 81mg; Sodium: 411mg; Carbohydrates: 56g; Fiber: 7g; Sugar: 3g; Protein: 33g

Turkey Cabbage Burgers

Prep time: 10 minutes   Cook time: 15 minutes

SERVES 4

NUT-FREE

Turkey burgers are a great way to enjoy an American favorite and stay solid on the MIND diet. Ground turkey is moist and flavorful and takes on the brightness of red bell pepper in this preparation. Turkey is a great source of the antioxidant mineral selenium, vitamin B_6, zinc, and phosphorus. Serve on a bun with your favorite condiments.

2 tablespoons olive oil

1 pound lean
   ground turkey

1 red bell pepper, minced

1 cup minced
   red cabbage

¼ cup bread crumbs

½ teaspoon dried
   thyme or ¼ teaspoon
   ground thyme

½ teaspoon dried
   rosemary

1. In a large pan or skillet, heat the olive oil over medium heat until shimmering.

2. While the oil is heating, in a large bowl, combine the turkey, bell pepper, cabbage, bread crumbs, thyme, and rosemary until all ingredients are well incorporated.

3. Split the mixture into quarters and shape into four patties.

4. Cook the patties for 5 to 7 minutes, flip, and cook the other side for 5 to 7 minutes, until cooked through and a meat thermometer reads 165°F.

> **Did you know?** Red cabbage contains higher amounts of key antioxidants and carotenoids than green cabbage due to the anthocyanins in the purple coloring.

Per serving (without bun): Calories: 263; Total fat: 15g; Saturated fat: 3.5g; Cholesterol: 81mg; Sodium: 131mg; Carbohydrates: 8g; Fiber: 1.5g; Sugar: 2.5g; Protein: 24g

Burrito Skillet

Prep time: 5 minutes   Cook time: 25 minutes
SERVES 4
GLUTEN-FREE NUT-FREE ONE-POT

This dish is like dinnertime chilaquiles. If you don't have tortillas in the pantry, this quick tortilla chip-topped skillet is the perfect alternative to satisfy your burrito craving. It all cooks in one skillet for an easy, filling meal with little cleanup on a busy weeknight.

1 tablespoon olive oil

1 pound lean
    ground turkey

2 cups crushed corn
    tortilla chips

1 (15-ounce) can no-salt-
    added black or pinto
    beans, drained

1 (14.5-ounce) can
    no-salt-added
    fire-roasted
    tomatoes, drained

½ tablespoon chili powder

½ teaspoon garlic powder

½ teaspoon onion powder

⅛ teaspoon
    cayenne pepper

1 large avocado

1. In a large and deep pan or skillet, heat the olive oil over medium heat until shimmering. Add the ground turkey and cook for 15 minutes, or until browned and cooked through.

2. Add the corn chips, beans, tomatoes, chili powder, garlic powder, onion powder, and cayenne pepper to the turkey and mix well. Cover the pan and cook together for 10 minutes.

3. Serve topped with sliced avocado.

> **Ingredient tip:** Canned corn and green chiles both make delicious additions to this skillet. You can serve it with any fresh toppings you have on hand like onions, tomatoes, or lettuce.

Per serving: Calories: 445; Total fat: 20g; Saturated fat: 4g; Cholesterol: 81mg; Sodium: 179mg; Carbohydrates: 36g; Fiber: 11g; Sugar: 3.5g; Protein: 31g

Fajita Chicken

Prep time: 5 minutes   Cook time: 25 minutes

SERVES 4

GLUTEN-FREE NUT-FREE ONE-POT

Fajitas are a classic flavor combination that pairs juicy chicken with fresh bell peppers and onions. The best thing about them is that you can make fajitas right at home, for cheaper than a restaurant, completely customizable to your liking.

1 pound boneless, skinless chicken breast

4 bell peppers, cut into strips (I prefer one of each color: red, orange, yellow, and green)

1 large onion, cut into strips

2 tablespoons olive oil

1 teaspoon chili powder

1 teaspoon ground cumin

1 teaspoon paprika

1. Preheat the oven to 400°F.
2. In a 9-by-12-inch baking dish, combine the chicken, bell peppers, and onion. Drizzle with the olive oil and sprinkle with the chili powder, cumin, and paprika. Cover with foil.
3. Bake for 20 to 25 minutes, or until the chicken reaches an internal temperature of 165°F and the juices run clear.

Variation tip: Enjoy this fajita chicken on its own or in tortillas, or use leftovers for a delicious breakfast.

Per serving: Calories: 251; Total fat: 10g; Saturated fat: 1.5g; Cholesterol: 83mg; Sodium: 57mg; Carbohydrates: 13g; Fiber: 2.5g; Sugar: 6g; Protein: 27g

One-Pan Tuscan Chicken

Prep time: 5 minutes   Cook time: 20 minutes
SERVES 4
GLUTEN-FREE NUT-FREE ONE-POT

Many dishes originating in Tuscany, Italy, feature fresh, simple ingredients and use olive oil instead of heavy sauces or butter. This chicken dish is a one-pot wonder full of bright flavors ready for your dinner table.

2 tablespoons olive oil

1 pound boneless, skinless chicken breast, cubed

1 cup cherry tomatoes, halved

1 cup fresh or frozen spinach

1 cup diced asparagus

½ cup low-sodium chicken stock

1 tablespoon white wine vinegar

1 tablespoon lemon juice

1 teaspoon dried rosemary

1 teaspoon dried or rubbed sage

1. In a large, deep pan or skillet, heat the olive oil over medium heat until shimmering. Cook the chicken for 5 to 7 minutes, until opaque and cooked through.

2. Add the tomatoes, spinach, asparagus, chicken stock, vinegar, lemon juice, rosemary, and sage and cook together for 5 to 10 more minutes, until the vegetables are tender.

Variation tip: This preparation would also work well with fish or shrimp.

Per serving: Calories: 210; Total fat: 10g; Saturated fat: 1.5g; Cholesterol: 83mg; Sodium: 73mg; Carbohydrates: 3g; Fiber: 1g; Sugar: 1g; Protein: 27g

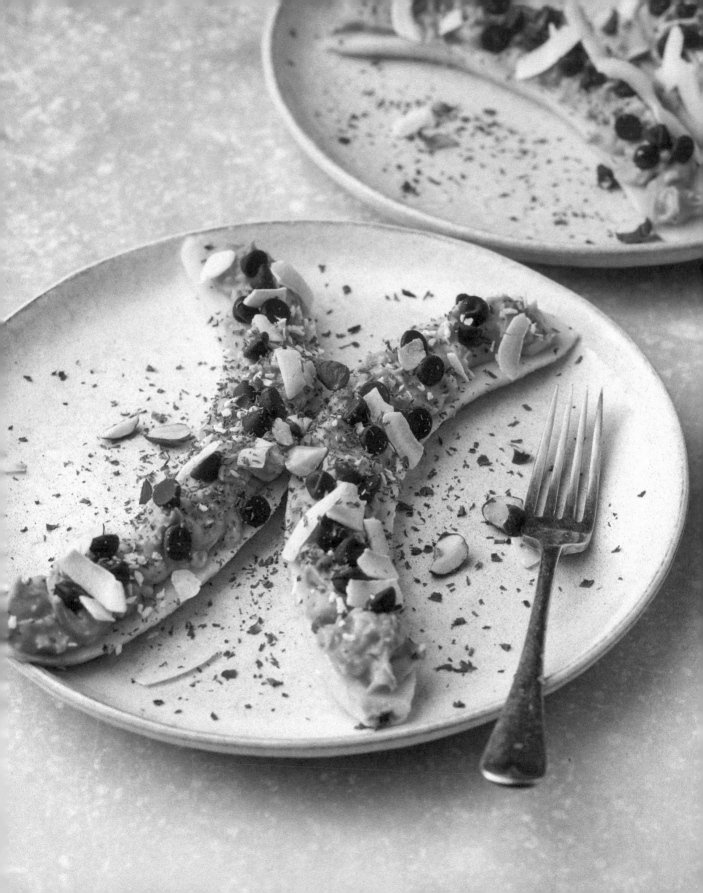

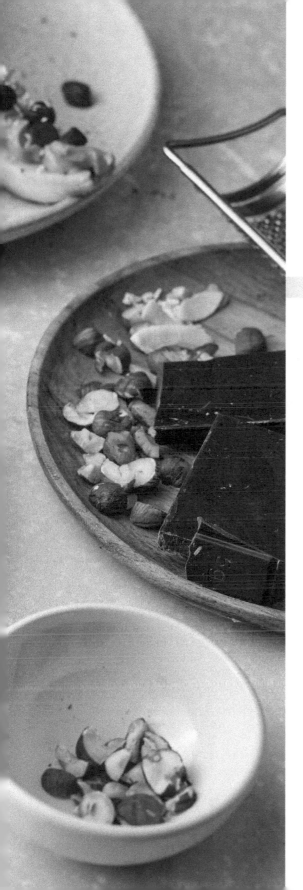

CHAPTER NINE

Sweet Treats

Banana Boats

Prep time: 5 minutes, plus 25 minutes in the freezer

SERVES 4

GLUTEN-FREE   ONE-POT   VEGAN

Do you remember ants on a log: celery with peanut butter and raisins? Meet the grown-up, MIND diet version: Banana Boats! This easy treat features frozen bananas topped with peanut butter and dark chocolate chips.

2 bananas

4 tablespoons crunchy peanut butter

2 tablespoons dark chocolate chips

1. Cut each banana in half lengthwise.

2. Spread each banana half with 1 tablespoon of peanut butter and sprinkle with ½ tablespoon of chocolate chips.

3. On a plate or tray, freeze the banana boats for 20 to 25 minutes before serving.

Did you know? Dark chocolate contains antioxidants including flavonols and polyphenols, both of which have proven effective at combating free radicals and preventing oxidative damage.

Per serving: Calories: 193; Total fat: 11g; Saturated fat: 3g; Cholesterol: 0mg; Sodium: 58mg; Carbohydrates: 21g; Fiber: 3.5g; Sugar: 11g; Protein: 5g

Berry Sorbet

Prep time: 5 minutes
SERVES 4
GLUTEN-FREE NUT-FREE ONE-POT VEGAN

Sorbet is a dairy-free alternative to ice cream that is also basically a frozen smoothie. Decreasing the liquid in any of your favorite smoothie recipes will yield sorbet. Make large batches of this berry-forward sorbet to keep in the freezer for a refreshing and nutritious treat.

1 cup frozen strawberries

1 cup frozen raspberries, blueberries, or blackberries (or a mix)

2 cups frozen peaches or bananas

2 tablespoons lime juice

1. Add the strawberries, raspberries, peaches, and lime juice to a blender and process on high for 30 to 60 seconds until no lumps remain.

2. Serve immediately or freeze.

> **Variation tip:** You can use any frozen fruit and blend it into sorbet. Use anything you have on hand or anything that you are craving.

Per serving: Calories. 48; Total fat: 0g; Saturated fat: 0g; Cholesterol: 0mg; Sodium: 1mg; Carbohydrates: 12g; Fiber: 2g; Sugar: 8g; Protein: 1g

Dark Chocolate–Covered Berries

Prep time: 10 minutes   Cook time: 5 minutes

SERVES 4

GLUTEN-FREE   NUT-FREE   VEGAN

Chocolate-covered fruit is no longer reserved for anniversaries or fine dining experiences. You can enjoy this decadent, healthy treat anytime from the comfort of your home.

1 cup dark chocolate chips

2 cups fresh berries of choice

1. Place the chocolate chips in a microwave-safe bowl and microwave for 2 minutes. Take the bowl out of the microwave to stir every 20 seconds to prevent burning. If the chocolate is fully melted before the 2 minutes are up, you can stop to prevent burning.

2. Add the berries to the melted chocolate and stir until well coated.

3. Using a slotted spoon, remove the berries from the bowl and place on a plate or tray lined with wax paper.

4. Freeze the berries for 5 minutes before serving.

Variation tip: Enjoy any fruit in this preparation. You can also freeze them completely for a frozen treat.

Per serving: Calories: 362; Total fat: 20g; Saturated fat: 12g; Cholesterol: 0mg; Sodium: 1mg; Carbohydrates: 43g; Fiber: 5.5g; Sugar: 31g; Protein: 5g

Peanut Butter Cups

Prep time: 10 minutes, plus freezing overnight
MAKES 6 CUPS
GLUTEN-FREE VEGAN

The only dessert simpler than this one is fruit—no kidding. Three ingredients and a freezer are all you need for a creamy, luscious, salty, sweet treat.

1½ cups creamy
   peanut butter
6 tablespoons fruit
   preserves of choice
½ teaspoon salt

1. Line a 6-cup cupcake tin with cupcake liners.
2. Scoop 2 tablespoons of peanut butter into the bottom of each cup, flattening with the back of a spoon to reach all edges.
3. Scoop 1 tablespoon of preserves into the center of each well.
4. Cover the preserves with 2 tablespoons of peanut butter per well, smoothing to reach all edges.
5. Sprinkle the cups with salt.
6. Freeze overnight and enjoy!

Did you know? The average American eats over 20 pounds of candy per year. Excess added sugar is not beneficial to brain health. Replace candy with treats like these peanut butter cups to reduce your consumption of added sugar.

Per serving (1 peanut butter cup): Calories. 433; Total fat: 33g; Saturated fat: 6.5g; Cholesterol: 0mg; Sodium: 466mg, Carbohydrates: 27g; Fiber: 3g; Sugar: 19g; Protein: 14g

Candied Dried Fruit

Prep time: 15 minutes   Cook time: 10 minutes

SERVES 4

GLUTEN-FREE NUT-FREE **VEGETARIAN**

Traditionally, making candied fruit requires knowledge of sugar temperatures and use of a candy thermometer. This recipe takes a lot of the guesswork out of it by using pre-dried fruit and simplifying the candying process.

¾ cup water

¼ cup honey

2 cups dried fruit
  of choice

1. In a large pot, bring the water and honey to a low boil over medium-high heat.

2. Remove the pot from the heat, add the dried fruit, and mix.

3. Soak the fruit in the sugar water for 5 minutes.

4. Remove the dried fruit from the pot using a slotted spoon and place on a cooling or drying rack for 10 minutes.

5. Store in an airtight container at room temperature or in the refrigerator for a cold, chewy treat.

Did you know? Dried fruit contains the same nutrients as fresh fruit. Because dried fruits shrink when they are dehydrated, you can eat a smaller volume than you would of fresh fruit while still getting all the same health benefits.

Per serving: Calories: 216; Total fat: 0g; Saturated fat: 0g; Cholesterol: 0mg; Sodium: 0mg; Carbohydrates: 56g; Fiber: 6g; Sugar: 48g; Protein: 2g

Cinnamon Roll Apples

Prep time: 10 minutes   Cook time: 10 minutes

SERVES 4

GLUTEN-FREE NUT-FREE ONE-POT VEGETARIAN

I can barely resist a fresh-baked cinnamon roll. Ooey-gooey dough and frosting take me straight home. Cinnamon rolls, unfortunately, are not exactly brain protective. These cinnamon roll apples, on the other hand, will satisfy your sweet tooth while benefiting your brain health.

2 pounds apples, sliced

¼ cup honey

2 tablespoons water

1 tablespoon olive oil

1 teaspoon ground cinnamon

½ teaspoon ground ginger

1. In a large microwave-safe bowl, combine the apples, honey, water, olive oil, cinnamon, and ginger and mix until the apples are well coated.

2. Microwave, covered with a splatter cover, for 6 to 8 minutes, until the apples are tender and the liquid is bubbling.

3. Let cool for 5 minutes before serving.

Variation tip: These apples make a delicious topping on oatmeal, cereal, waffles, pancakes, or even fruit sorbet.

Per serving. Calories: 201; Total fat: 3.5g; Saturated fat: 0.5g; Cholesterol: 0mg; Sodium: 3mg; Carbohydrates: 46g; Fiber: 5g; Sugar: 38g; Protein: 1g

Cereal Clusters

Prep time: 20 minutes
SERVES 4
VEGETARIAN

These rich, satisfying clusters are great for dessert but can also be enjoyed as a midday snack or even for breakfast. They are proof that sometimes combining the simplest ingredients, like peanut butter, honey, and a crunchy cereal, yields the tastiest results!

2 cups whole-grain cereal

½ cup creamy peanut butter

1 tablespoon honey

½ teaspoon ground cinnamon

1. In a large bowl, combine the cereal, peanut butter, honey, and cinnamon and mix until the cereal is well coated.

2. On a plate or tray lined with wax paper, drop the cereal in clusters about 2 tablespoons in size.

3. Freeze for 15 minutes before serving.

Substitution tip: Make these treats gluten-free by substituting your favorite gluten-free cereal.

Per serving: Calories: 252; Total fat: 17g; Saturated fat: 3.5g; Cholesterol: 0mg; Sodium: 181mg; Carbohydrates: 20g; Fiber: 1.5g; Sugar: 8g; Protein: 9g

Peanut Butter Cookies

Prep time: 10 minutes   Cook time: 15 minutes
MAKES 2 DOZEN COOKIES
VEGETARIAN

Wouldn't it be great if dessert also gave you a nice boost of protein? Thank goodness for peanut butter cookies! Creamy peanut butter is high in protein and contains key vitamins and minerals to promote brain health.

1 cup whole wheat flour

1 teaspoon baking soda

¼ teaspoon salt

1 cup creamy peanut butter

½ cup honey

⅓ cup plain unsweetened nondairy milk

1 teaspoon vanilla extract

1. Preheat the oven to 350°F. Line two baking sheets with parchment paper and set aside.

2. In a large bowl, whisk together the flour, baking soda, and salt until all ingredients are well combined. In a second bowl, stir together the peanut butter, honey, nondairy milk, and vanilla until all ingredients are well combined.

3. Add the wet ingredients to the dry ingredients and mix with clean or gloved hands. The dough will be too stiff to mix with a spoon. Knead the dough until there are no patches of dry ingredients remaining.

4. Make 24 balls, each with 1 heaping tablespoon of dough. Place each ball at least 1 inch apart on the prepared baking sheets. Using the back of a fork, flatten each cookie in a crisscross pattern.

5. Bake the cookies for 10 minutes for a chewy texture or 12 to 13 minutes for crispier cookies.

6. Serve warm or cooled.

Cooking tip: These cookies freeze well for up to 60 days.

Per serving (2 cookies): Calories: 206; Total fat: 11g; Saturated fat: 2g; Cholesterol: 0mg; Sodium: 250mg; Carbohydrates: 24g; Fiber: 2g; Sugar: 14g; Protein: 6g

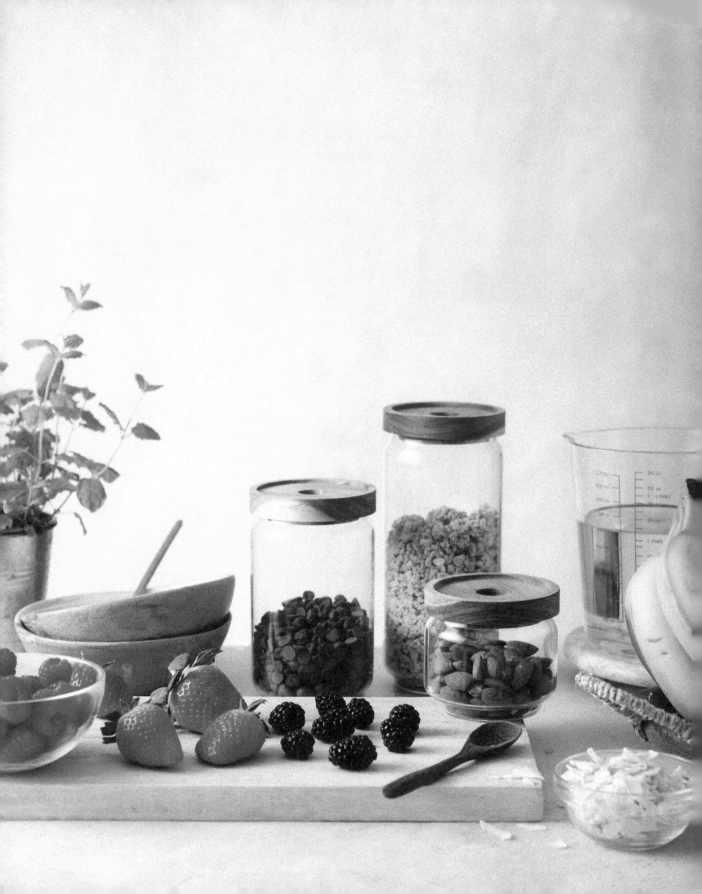

MEASUREMENT CONVERSIONS

	US STANDARD	US STANDARD (OUNCES)	METRIC (APPROXIMATE)
VOLUME EQUIVALENTS (LIQUID)	2 tablespoons	1 fl. oz.	30 mL
	¼ cup	2 fl. oz.	60 mL
	½ cup	4 fl. oz.	120 mL
	1 cup	8 fl. oz.	240 mL
	1½ cups	12 fl. oz.	355 mL
	2 cups or 1 pint	16 fl. oz.	475 mL
	4 cups or 1 quart	32 fl. oz.	1 L
	1 gallon	128 fl. oz.	4 L
VOLUME EQUIVALENTS (DRY)	⅛ teaspoon		0.5 mL
	¼ teaspoon		1 mL
	½ teaspoon		2 mL
	¾ teaspoon		4 mL
	1 teaspoon		5 mL
	1 tablespoon		15 mL
	¼ cup		59 mL
	⅓ cup		79 mL
	½ cup		118 mL
	⅔ cup		156 mL
	¾ cup		177 mL
	1 cup		235 mL
	2 cups or 1 pint		475 mL
	3 cups		700 mL
	4 cups or 1 quart		1 L
	½ gallon		2 L
	1 gallon		4 L
WEIGHT EQUIVALENTS	½ ounce		15 g
	1 ounce		30 g
	2 ounces		60 g
	4 ounces		115 g
	8 ounces		225 g
	12 ounces		340 g
	16 ounces or 1 pound		455 g

	FAHRENHEIT (F)	CELSIUS (C) (APPROXIMATE)
OVEN TEMPERATURES	250°F	120°C
	300°F	150°C
	325°F	180°C
	375°F	190°C
	400°F	200°C
	425°F	220°C
	450°F	230°C

RESOURCES

Check out these resources for more information on eating to promote brain health.

Diet for the MIND **by Martha Morris:** When searching for answers about the MIND diet, you can always go straight to the expert source, Dr. Morris's book.

Alz.org: From facts to research and from support to local resources, the Alzheimer's Association website has an abundance of information about cognitive decline.

Eatright.org: This site features practical, real-life nutrition tips for any and everyone, including for the MIND diet.

Jandonline.org: Peer-reviewed studies and research from the *Journal of the Academy of Nutrition and Dietetics* are all available at your fingertips.

Rush.edu: Dr. Morris performed her research through Rush University Medical Center, and its site has a wealth of information on cognitive decline and the MIND diet.

REFERENCES

Alzheimer's Association. "Facts and Figures." Accessed September 21, 2020. alz.org/alzheimers-dementia/facts-figures#:~:text=One%20in%2010%20people%20age,other%20dementias%20as%20older%20whites.

Alzheimer's Association. "Mild Cognitive Impairment (MCI)." Accessed September 21, 2020. alz.org/alzheimers-dementia/what-is-dementia/related_conditions/mild-cognitive-impairment.

Alzheimer's Association. "Reducing Stress." Accessed September 21, 2020. alz.org/help-support/i-have-alz/live-well/reducing-stress.

Barnes, Jennifer L., Min Tian, Neile K. Edens, and Martha Clare Morris. "Consideration of Nutrient Levels in Studies of Cognitive Decline." *Nutrition Reviews* 72, no. 11 (November 2014): 707–19. doi.org/10.1111/nure.12144.

Barnes, Jill N. "Exercise, Cognitive Function, and Aging." *Advances in Physiology Education* 39, no. 2 (June 2015): 55–62. doi.org/10.1152/advan.00101.2014.

Bennett, David A., Julie A. Schneider, Aron S. Buchman, Lisa L. Barnes, Patricia A. Boyle, and Robert S. Wilson. "Overview and Findings from the Rush Memory and Aging Project." *Current Alzheimer Research* 9, no. 6 (2012): 646–63. doi.org/10.2174/156720512801322663.

Calon, Frédéric, Giselle P. Lim, Fusheng Yang, Takashi Morihara, Bruce Teter, Oliver Ubeda, Phillippe Rostaing, Antoine Triller, Norman Salem Jr., Karen H. Ashe, Sally A. Frautschy, and Greg M. Cole. "Docosahexaenoic Acid Protects from Dendritic Pathology in an Alzheimer's Disease Mouse Model." *Neuron* 43, no. 5 (September 2004): 633–45. doi.org/10.1016/j.neuron.2004.08.013.

Chen, X., Yuegin Huang, and H. G. Cheng. "Lower Intake of Vegetables and Legumes Associated with Cognitive Decline among Illiterate Elderly Chinese: A 3-Year Cohort Study." *Journal of Nutrition, Health & Aging* 16 (February 2012): 549–52. doi.org/10.1007/s12603-012-0023-2.

Devore, Elizabeth E., Jae Hee Kang, Monique M. B. Breteler, and Francine Grodstein. "Dietary Intakes of Berries and Flavonoids in Relation to Cognitive Decline." *Annals of Neurology* 72, no. 1 (April 2012): 135–43. doi.org/10.1002/ana.23594.

Ellingsworth, Christy, and Murdoc Khaleghi. *The Everything Guide to the MIND Diet.* Avon: Adams Media, 2016.

Féart, Catherine, Cécilia Samieri, and Virginie Rondeau. "Adherence to a Mediterranean Diet, Cognitive Decline, and Risk of Dementia." *Journal of the American Medical Association* 302, no. 6 (August 2009): 638–48. doi.org/10.1001/jama.2009.1146.

Harvard Medical School. "How Can You Prevent Cognitive Decline? Try This Combination Strategy." Accessed September 21, 2020. health.harvard .edu/mind-and-mood/how-can-you-prevent-cognitive-decline-try-this -combination-strategy.

Harvard Medical School. "Protecting against Cognitive Decline." Accessed September 21, 2020. health.harvard.edu/mind-and-mood/protecting -against-cognitive-decline.

Janson, Juliette, Thomas Laedtke, Joseph E. Parisi, Peter O'Brien, Ronald C. Petersen, and Peter C. Butler. "Increased Risk of Type 2 Diabetes in Alzheimer Disease." *Diabetes* 53, no. 2 (February 2004): 474–81. doi.org/10.2337/diabetes.53.2.474.

Joseph, J. A., G. Arendash, M. Gordon, D. Diamond, B. Shukitt-Hale, D. Morgan, and N. A. Denisova. "Blueberry Supplementation Enhances Signaling and Prevents Behavioral Deficits in an Alzheimer Disease Model." *Nutritional Neuroscience* 6, no. 3 (2003): 153–62. doi.org/10.1080/1028415031000111282.

Joseph, James A., Barbara Shukitt-Hale, Natalia A. Denisova, Donna Bielinksi, Antonio Martin, John J. McEwen, and Paula C. Bickford. "Reversals of Age-Related Declines in Neuronal Signal Transduction, Cognitive, and Motor Behavioral Deficits with Blueberry, Spinach, or Strawberry Dietary Supplementation." *Journal of Neuroscience* 19, no. 18 (September 1999): 8114–21. doi.org/10.1523/JNEUROSCI.19-18-08114.1999.

Kalmijn, Sandra, Lenore J. Launer, Alewijn Ott, Jacqueline C. Witteman, Albert Hofman, and Monique M. B. Breteler. "Dietary Fat Intake and the Risk of Incident Dementia in the Rotterdam Study." *Annals of Neurology* 42, no. 5 (November 1997): 776–82. doi.org/10.1002/ana.410420514.

Kang, Jae H., Alberto Ascherio, and Francine Grodstein. "Fruit and Vegetable Consumption and Cognitive Decline in Aging Women." *Annals of Neurology* 57, no. 5 (May 2005): 713–20. doi.org/10.1002/ana.20476.

Lim, G. P., F. Calon, T. Morihara, F. Yang, B. Teter, O. Ubeda, N. Salem, Jr., S. A. Frautschy, and G. M. Cole. "A Diet Enriched with the Omega-3 Fatty Acid Docosahexaenoic Acid Reduces Amyloid Burden in an Aged Alzheimer Mouse Model." *Journal of Neuroscience* 25, no. 12 (March 2005): 3032–40. doi.org/10.1523/JNEUROSCI.4225-04.2005.

Marcason, Wendy. "What Are the Components to the MIND Diet?" *Journal of the Academy of Nutrition and Dietetics* 115, no. 10 (October 2015): 1744. doi.org/10.1016/j.jand.2015.08.002.

Martinez-Lapiscina, Elena H., Pedro Clavero, Estefania Toledo, Ramon Estruch, Jordi Salas-Salvado, Beatriz San Julian, Ana Sanchez-Tainta, Emilio Ros, Cinta Valls-Pedret, and Miguel A. Martinez-Gonzalez. "Mediterranean Diet Improves Cognition: The PREDIMED-NAVARRA Randomised Trial." *Journal of Neurology, Neurosurgery, and Psychiatry* 84, no. 12 (December 2013): 1318–25. doi.org/10.1136/jnnp-2012-304792?

Morris, Martha. *Diet for the MIND: The Latest Science for What to Eat to Prevent Alzheimer's and Cognitive Decline*. New York: Hachette Book Group, 2017.

Morris, Martha. "Nutritional Determinants of Cognitive Aging and Dementia." *Proceedings of Nutrition Society* 71, no. 1 (2011): 1–13. doi.org/10.1017/S0029665111003296.

Morris, Martha C. "The Role of Nutrition in Alzheimer's Disease: Epidemiological Evidence." *European Journal of Neurology* 16, supp. 1 (September 2009): 1–7. doi.org/10.1111/j.1468-1331.2009.02735.x.

Morris, Martha, and Christy C. Tangney. "Dietary Fat Composition and Dementia Risk." *Neurobiology of Aging* 35, supp. 2 (September 2014): S59–S62. doi.org/10.1016/j.neurobiolaging.2014.03.038.

Morris, Martha, Christy C. Tangney, Yamin Wang, Lisa L. Barnes, David Bennett, and Neelum Aggarwal. "MIND Diet Score More Predictive Than DASH or Mediterranean Diet Scores." *Alzheimer's Association International Conference* (July 2014): 166. doi.org/10.1016/j.jalz.2014.04.164.

Morris, Martha, Christy C. Tangney, Yamin Wang, Frank M. Sacks, Lisa L. Barnes, David A. Bennett, and Neelum T. Aggarwal. "MIND Diet Slows Cognitive Decline with Aging." *Alzheimer's & Dementia* 11, no. 9 (September 2015): 1015–22. doi.org/10.1016/j.jalz.2015.04.011.

Morris, Martha, Christy C. Tangney, Yamin Wang, Frank M. Sacks, David A. Bennett, and Neelum T. Aggarwal. "MIND Diet Associated with Reduced Incidence of Alzheimer's Disease." *Alzheimer's & Dementia* 11, no. 9 (September 2015): 1007–14. doi.org/10.1016/j.jalz.2014.11.009.

Morris, Martha, D. A. Evans, Christy C. Tangney, J. L. Bienias, and R. S. Wilson. "Associations of Vegetable and Fruit Consumption with Age-Related Cognitive Change." *Neurology* 67, no. 8 (October 2006): 1370–76. doi.org/10.1212/01.wnl.0000240224.38978.d8.

Morris, Martha, Denis A. Evans, Christy C. Tangney, Julia L. Bienias, and Robert S. Wilson. "Fish Consumption and Cognitive Decline with Age in a Large Community Study." *Archives of Neurology* 62, no. 12 (2005): 1849–53. doi.org/10.1001/archneur.62.12.noc50161.

Morris, Martha, Christy C. Tangney, Yamin Wang, Frank M. Sacks, David A. Bennett, and Neelum T. Aggarwal. "MIND Diet Associated with Reduced Incidence of Alzheimer's Disease." *Alzheimer's & Dementia* 11, no. 9 (September 2015): 1007–14. doi.org/10.1016/j.jalz.2014.11.009.

Morris, Martha, Denis A. Evans, Julia L. Bienias, Christine C. Tangney, David A. Bennett, Robert S. Wilson, Neelum Aggarwal, and Julie Schneider. "Consumption of Fish and N-3 Fatty Acids and Risk of Incident Alzheimer Disease." *Archives of Neurology* 60, no. 7 (2003): 940–46. doi.org/10.1001/archneur.60.7.940

Nishida, Yoichiro, Shingo Ito, Sumio Ohtsuki, Naoki Yamamoto, Tsubura Takahashi, Nobuhisa Iwata, Kou-ichi Jishage, et al. "Depletion of Vitamin E Increases Amyloid Beta Accumulation by Decreasing Its Clearances from Brain and Blood in a Mouse Model of Alzheimer Disease." *Journal of Biological Chemistry* 284, no. 48 (November 2009): 33400–33408. doi.org/10.1074/jbc.M109.054056.

Nooyens, Astrid C. J., H. Bas Bueno-de-Mesquita, Martin P. J. van Boxtel, Boukje M. van Gelder, Hans Verhagen, and W. M. Monique Verschuren. "Fruit and Vegetable Intake and Cognitive Decline in Middle-Aged Men and Women: The Doetinchem Cohort Study." *British Journal of Nutrition* 106, no. 5 (September 2011): 752–61. doi.org/10.1017/S0007114511001024.

Obulesu, M., Muralidhara Rao Dowlathabad, and P. V. Bramhachari. "Carotenoids and Alzheimer's Disease: An Insight into Therapeutic Role of Retinoids in Animal Models." *Neurochemistry International* 59, no. 5 (October 2011): 535–41. doi.org/10.1016/j.neuint.2011.04.004.

Roberts, Rosebud O., Yonus E. Geda, James R. Cerhan, David S. Knopman, Ruth H. Cha, Teresa J. H. Christianson, V. Shane Pankratz, Robert J. Ivnik, Bradley F. Boeve, Helen M. O'Connor, and Ronald C. Petersen. "Vegetables, Unsaturated Fats, Moderate Alcohol Intake, and Mild Cognitive Impairment." *Dementia and Geriatric Cognitive Disorders* 29, no. 5 (June 2010): 413–23. doi.org/10.1159/000305099.

Rush University Medical Center. "Diet May Help Prevent Alzheimer's: MIND Diet Rich in Vegetables, Berries, Whole Grains, Nuts." Accessed September 21, 2020. rush.edu/news/diet-may-help-prevent-alzheimers.

Scarmeas, Nikolaos, Yaakov Stern, Ming-Xin Tang, Richard Mayeux, and Jose A. Luchsinger. "Mediterranean Diet and Risk for Alzheimer's Disease." *Annals of Neurology* 56, no. 6 (June 2006): 912–21. doi.org/10.1002/ana.20854.

Spira, Adam P., Lenis P. Chen-Edinboro, Mark N. Wu, and Kristine Yaffe. "Impact of Sleep on the Risk of Cognitive Decline and Dementia." *Current Opinion in Psychiatry* 27, no. 6 (November 2014): 478–83. doi.org/10.1097/YCO.0000000000000106.

Tangney, Christy C., Hong Li, Yamin Wang, Lisa Barnes, Julie A. Schneider, David A. Bennett, and Martha C. Morris. "Relation of DASH- and Mediterranean-Like Dietary Patterns to Cognitive Decline in Older Persons." *Neurology* 83, no. 16 (October 2014): 1410–16. doi.org/10.1212/wnl.0000000000000884.

Tangney, Christine C., Mary J. Kwasny, Hong Li, Robert S. Wilson, Denis A. Evans, and Martha C. Morris. "Adherence to a Mediterranean-Type Dietary Pattern and Cognitive Decline in a Community Population." *American Journal of Clinical Nutrition* 93, no. 3 (March 2011): 601–7. doi.org/10.3945/ajcn.110.007369.

Tangney, Christine C., Hong Li, Lisa L. Barnes, Julie A. Schneider, David A. Bennett, and Martha C. Morris. "Accordance to Dietary Approaches to Stop Hypertension (DASH) Is Associated with Slower Cognitive Decline." *Alzheimer's & Dementia* 9, no. 4S (July 2013): 605–6. doi.org/10.1016/j.jalz.2013.04.075.

Tsivgoulis, Georgios, Suzanne Judd, Abraham J. Letter, Andrei V. Alexandrov, George Howard, Fadi Nahab, Frederick W. Unverzagt, Claudia Moy, Virginia J. Howard, Brett Kissela, and Virginia G. Wadley. "Adherence to a Mediterranean Diet and Risk of Incident Cognitive Impairment." *Neurology* 80, no. 18 (April 2013): 1684–92. doi.org/10.1212/WNL.0b013e3182904f69.

Van de Rest, Ondine, Agnes A. Berendsen, Annemien Haveman-Niles, and Lisette C. de Groot. "Dietary Patterns, Cognitive Decline, and Dementia: A Systematic Review." *Advances in Nutrition* 6, no. 2 (March 2015): 154–68. doi.org/10.3945/an.114.007617.

Wengreen, Heidi, Ronald G. Munger, Adele Cutler, Anna Quach, Austin Bowles, Christopher Corcoran, JoAnn T. Tschanz, Maria C. Norton, and Kathleen A. Welsh-Bohmer. "Prospective Study of Dietary Approaches to Stop Hypertension and Mediterranean-Style Dietary Patterns and Age-Related Cognitive Change: The Cache County Study on Memory, Health and Aging." *American Journal of Clinical Nutrition* 98, no. 5 (November 2013): 1263–71. doi.org/10.3945/ajcn.112.051276.

Willis, Lauren, Barbara Shukitt-Hale, and James A. Joseph. "Recent Advances in Berry Supplementation and Age-Related Cognitive Decline." *Current Opinion in Clinical Nutrition and Metabolic Care* 12, no. 1 (January 2009): 91–94. doi.org/10.1097/MCO.0b013e32831b9c6e.

Wingo, Thomas S., David J. Cutler, Aliza P. Wingo, Ngoc-Anh Le, Gil D. Rabinovici, Bruce L. Miller, James J. Lah, and Allan I. Levey. "Association of Early-Onset Alzheimer Disease with Elevated Low-Density Lipoprotein Cholesterol Levels and Rare Genetic Coding Variants of *APOB*." *JAMA Neurology* 76, no. 7 (May 2019): 807–17. doi.org/10.1001/jamaneurol.2019.0648.

INDEX

ACKNOWLEDGMENTS

Thank you to my husband, family, friends, and colleagues, whose unwavering support pushed me through the long nights writing. Thank you to the incredible team at Callisto. Without your hard work behind the scenes, none of these books would ever reach the shelves.

ABOUT THE AUTHOR

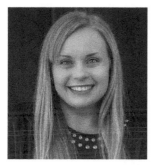 **Amanda Foote, RD,** is a registered dietitian, proud fire wife, and mother. She runs her own virtual nutrition practice, Amanda Foote Nutrition, specializing in intuitive eating and food freedom. It is her calling to ensure that food remains an enjoyable, nourishing part of the human experience.

Amanda has previously worked as a registered dietitian for InnovAge and South Adams County Fire Department. Amanda has a bachelor's degree in dietetics from the University of Northern Colorado, and a bachelor's degree in applied psychology from Regis University.

Amanda lives in Colorado with her family and pets. In her spare time, she enjoys developing new recipes, sketching, reading, and camping.

CPSIA information can be obtained
at www.ICGtesting.com
Printed in the USA
BVHW091655310821
615706BV00012B/191